Acta Hæmatologica

Founded 1948 by E. Meulengracht, K. Rohr, and G. Rosenow
Continued by H. Lüdin (1960–1977), U. Bucher (1977–1983), R.S. Hillman (1978–1987),
H.R. Marti (1983–1988), E.A. Beck (1984–1988), B. Ramot (1989–1995)

KARGER

Printed in Switzerland
on acid-free and non-aging
paper (ISO 9706) by
Reinhardt Druck, Basel

Appears 6-weekly:
2 volumes per year
(8 issues)

Guidelines for Authors

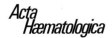

Submission

Manuscripts written in English should be submitted using the online submission website at:

www.karger.com/aha

or as an e-mail attachment (the preferred word-processing package is MS-Word) to the Editorial Office:

aha@karger.ch

Prof. I. Ben-Bassat
S. KARGER AG
Editorial Office 'Acta Haematologica'
PO Box
CH-4009 Basel (Switzerland)

All manuscripts must be accompanied by a covering letter signed by all authors. Assurance should be given that the manuscript is not under simultaneous consideration by any other publication. The preferred word processing package is Word for Windows®. Presentation of manuscripts should conform with the Uniform Requirements for Manuscripts Submitted to Biomedical Journals (see N Engl J Med 1997;336:309–315).

Conditions

All manuscripts are subject to editorial review. Manuscripts are received with the explicit understanding that they are not under simultaneous consideration by any other publication. Submission of an article for publication implies the transfer of the copyright from the author to the publisher upon acceptance. Accepted papers become the permanent property of 'Acta Haematologica' and may not be reproduced by any means, in whole or in part, without the written consent of the publisher. It is the author's responsibility to obtain permission to reproduce illustrations, tables, etc. from other publications.

Arrangement

Recommendation for Usage of Units and Abbreviations: The standard abbreviations used for measurements of weight, length, volume, and time (i.e. mg, cm, ml, min) are used without definition. The abbreviations listed on the opposite page also require no definition. Please note that punctuation is not needed. The usage of units as recommended in the table on the opposite page is required. When listed the alternative units can be used.

Title page: The first page of each paper should indicate the title, the authors' names, the institute where the work was conducted, and a short title for use as running head.
NB: Authors wishing to preserve the phonetic meaning of diacritics (PubMed reduces diacritics to their root characters) must spell their names accordingly when submitting manuscripts (e.g. Müller should be Mueller).

Full address: The exact postal address of the corresponding author complete with postal code must be given at the bottom of the title page. Please also supply phone and fax numbers, as well as e-mail address.

Key words: For indexing purposes, a list of 3–10 key words in English is essential.

Abstract: Each paper needs an abstract of up to 10 lines.

Footnotes: Avoid footnotes. When essential, they are numbered consecutively and typed at the foot of the appropriate page.

Tables and illustrations: Tables and illustrations (both numbered in Arabic numerals) should be prepared on separate sheets. Tables require a heading and figures a legend, also prepared on a separate sheet. For the reproduction of illustrations, only good drawings and original photographs can be accepted; negatives or photocopies cannot be used. Due to technical reasons, figures with a screen background should not be submitted. When possible, group several illustrations on one block for reproduction (max. size 180 × 223 mm) or provide crop marks. On the back of each illustration, indicate its number, the author's name, and 'top' with a soft pencil. Electronically submitted b/w half-tone and color illustrations must have a final resolution of 300 dpi after scaling, line drawings one of 800–1,200 dpi.

Color illustrations
Online edition: Color illustrations are reproduced free of charge. In the print version, the illustrations are reproduced in black and white. Please avoid referring to the colors in the text and figure legends.
Print edition: Up to 6 color illustrations per page can be integrated within the text at CHF 760.– per page.

References: In the text identify references by Arabic numerals [in square brackets]. Material submitted for publication but not yet accepted should be noted as 'unpublished data' and not be included in the reference list. The list of references should include only those publications which are cited in the text. Do not alphabetize; number references in the order in which they are first mentioned in the text. The surnames of the authors followed by initials should be given. There should be no punctuation other than a comma to separate the authors. Please cite all authors, 'et al' is not sufficient. Abbreviate journal names according to the Index Medicus system. (Also see International Committee of Medical Journal Editors: Uniform requirements for manuscripts submitted to biomedical journals. N Engl J Med 1997;336:309–315.)

Examples
(a) Papers published in periodicals: Sun J, Koto H, Chung KF: Interaction of ozone and allergen challenges on bronchial responsiveness and inflammation in sensitised guinea pigs. Int Arch Allergy Immunol 1997;112:191–195.
(b) Papers published only with DOI numbers: Theoharides TC, Boucher W, Spear K: Serum interleukin-6 reflects disease severity and osteoporosis in mastocytosis patients. Int Arch Allergy Immunol DOI: 10.1159/000063858.
(c) Monographs: Matthews DE, Farewell VT: Using and Understanding Medical Statistics, ed 3, revised. Basel, Karger, 1996.
(d) Edited books: Parren PWHI, Burton DR: Antibodies against HIV-1 from phage display libraries: Mapping of an immune response and progress towards antiviral immunotherapy; in Capra JD (ed): Antibody Engineering. Chem Immunol. Basel, Karger, 1997, vol 65, pp 18–56.

Reference Management Software: Use of EndNote is recommended for easy management and formatting of citations and reference lists.

Digital Object Identifier (DOI)

S. Karger Publishers supports DOIs as unique identifiers for articles. A DOI number will be printed on the title page of each article. DOIs can be useful in the future for identifying and citing articles published online without volume or issue information. More information can be found at www.doi.org.

Author's Choice™

With this option the author can choose to make his article freely available online against a one-time fee of CHF 2750.–. This fee is independent of any standard charges for supplementary pages, color images etc. which may apply. More information can be found at www.karger.com/authors_choice.

Page Charges

Authors are charged CHF 155.– per printed page for the first 6 pages and CHF 310.– for each additional page, including tables, illustrations, and references. 1 printed page is equal to approximately 3 manuscript pages.

Rapid Communication

Manuscripts intended for rapid communication must present new findings of sufficient importance to justify their accelerated acceptance. They should follow the general arrangement of research papers except that the separate sections should not be formally titled. They should not be more than three pages in length (including figures, tables and references). Proofs are checked by the Main Editor and not sent to the authors. Review will be rapid, and once accepted, the paper will be included in the next planned issue. If manuscripts require significant change after editing they will be treated as brief communications and returned to the authors for correction.

Brief Communication

The general arrangement for brief communications is the same as for research papers except that the manuscript is not divided into separate sections formally entitled introduction, methods, results, discussion. No abstract is required. These should not be more than 3 pages in length.

Letter to the Editor

Comments and responses to previously published articles and other short correspondences are welcome. They should be limited to 1 or 1¼ manuscript pages with a general arrangement as specified for Brief Communications.

Proofs

Unless indicated otherwise, proofs are sent to the first-named author and should be returned with the least possible delay. Alterations made in proofs, other than the correction of printer's errors, are charged to the author. No page proofs are supplied.

Reprints

Order forms and a price list are sent with the proofs. Orders submitted after the issue is printed are subject to considerably higher prices.

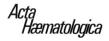
Usage of Units and Abbreviations

Entity	Abbreviation	Recommended unit	Alternative unit
Red blood cell count	RBC	$\times 10^{12}/l$	
White blood cell count	WBC	$\times 10^{9}/l$	
Platelet count	PLT	$\times 10^{9}/l$	
Reticulocyte count	RETIC	%	
Hemoglobin	Hb	g/dl	
Hematocrit (packed cell volume)	HCT	ratio, no unit necessary	
Mean cell volume	MCV	fl	
Mean cell hemoglobin	MCH	pg	
Mean cell hemoglobin concentration	MCHC	g/dl	
Sedimentation rate	ESR	mm/h	
Serum vitamin B_{12}		pg/ml	pmol/l
Serum folate		ng/ml	nmol/l
Serum iron		µg/dl	µmol/l
Iron-binding capacity	IBC	µg/dl	µmol/l
Serum ferritin		ng/ml	µg/l
Transferrin		mg/dl	g/l
Serum haptoglobin		mg/dl	g/l
Fibrinogen		mg/dl	g/l
Immunoglobulin G, A, M	IgG, IgA, IgM	mg/dl	g/l
Beta-2-microglobulin	β_2m	mg/l	

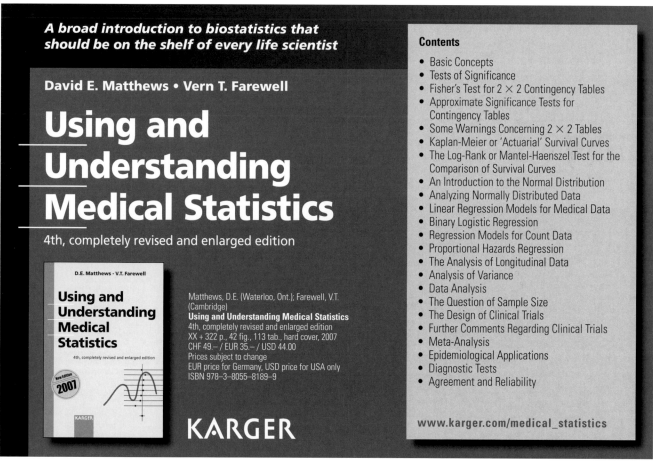
KARGER

© 2009 S. Karger AG, Basel

Fax +41 61 306 12 34
E-Mail karger@karger.ch
www.karger.com

The Guidelines for Authors are available at:
www.karger.com/aha_Guidelines

General Information

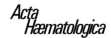

ISSN Print Edition: 0001–5792
ISSN Online Edition: 1421–9662

Journal Homepage: www.karger.com/aha

Publication Data: 'Acta Haematologica' is published 8 times a year. Volumes 121–122, each with 4 issues, appear in 2009.

Subscription Rates: Subscriptions run for a full calendar year. Prices are given per year.
Personal subscription:

Print or Online	Print+Online combined
CHF 1236.–	CHF 1326.–
EUR 883.–	EUR 947.–
USD 1177.00	USD 1263.00

postage and handling (added to print and print+online)
CHF 50.40 Europe, CHF 75.60 Overseas
EUR 36.–
USD 71.60

Institutional subscription:

Print or Online	Print+Online combined
CHF 2472.–	CHF 2720.–
EUR 1766.–	EUR 1942.–
USD 2354.00	USD 2590.00

postage and handling (added to print and print+online)
CHF 63.20 Europe, CHF 94.40 Overseas
EUR 44.80
USD 89.60
Airmail surcharge: CHF 64.– / USD 60.80
Discount subscription prices:
    International Society of Haematology

Back Volumes and Single Issues: Information on availability and prices of single print issues and print or electronic back volumes can be obtained from Customer Service at *service@karger.ch.*

Bibliographic Indices: This journal is regularly listed in bibliographic services, including *Current Contents*® and PubMed/MEDLINE.

Subscription Orders:
Orders can be placed at agencies, bookstores, directly with the Publisher

S. Karger AG
Medical and Scientific Publishers
P.O. Box
CH–4009 Basel
Switzerland
(for courier services only:
Allschwilerstrasse 10
CH–4055 Basel)
Tel. +41 61 306 11 11
Fax +41 61 306 12 34
E-Mail karger@karger.ch
www.karger.com

Change of Address:
Both old and new address should be sent to the subscription source.

or further Karger offices
or representatives:

France:
Librairie Medi-Sciences Sarl
36, bd de Latour-Maubourg
75007 Paris
France
Tél. +33 (0) 1 45 51 42 58
Fax +33 (0) 1 45 56 07 80
E-Mail librairie@medi-sciences.fr
www.medi-sciences.fr

Germany:
S. Karger GmbH
Postfach
79095 Freiburg
Deutschland
(Hausadresse: Lörracher Strasse 16A
79115 Freiburg)
Tel. +49 761 45 20 70
Fax +49 761 45 20 714
E-Post information@karger.de
www.karger.de

India, Bangladesh, Sri Lanka:
Panther Publishers Private Ltd.
33, First Main
Koramangala First Block
Bangalore 560 034
India
Tel. +91 80 25505 836
Tel. +91 80 25505 837
Fax +91 80 25505 981
E-Mail panther_publishers@vsnl.com
www.pantherpublishers.com

Japan:
Karger Japan, Inc.
Yushima S Bld. 3F
4-2-3, Yushima, Bunkyo-ku
Tokyo 113-0034
Japan
Tel. +81 3 3815 1800
Fax +81 3 3815 1802
E-Mail publisher@karger.jp

China, Taiwan and Malaysia:
Karger China
Suite 409, Apollo Building
1440 Central Yan An Road
Shanghai 200040
China
Tel. +86-21-6133 1861
Fax +86-21-6133 1862
E-Mail karger.ray@gmail.com

South America and Central America:
Cranbury International LLC
7 Clarendon Ave., Suite 2
Montpelier, VT 05602
USA
Tel. +1 802 223 6565
Fax +1 802 223 6824
E-Mail
eatkin@cranburyinternational.com
www.cranburyinternational.com

United Kingdom, Ireland:
S. Karger AG
c/o London Liaison Office
4 Rickett Street
London SW6 1RU
United Kingdom
Tel. +44 (0) 20 7386 0500
Fax +44 (0) 20 7610 3337
E-Mail uk@karger.ch

USA:
S. Karger Publishers, Inc.
26 West Avon Road
P.O. Box 529
Unionville, CT 06085
USA
Toll free: +1 800 828 5479
Tel. +1 860 675-7834
Fax +1 860 675-7302
E-Mail karger@snet.net

KARGER

© 2009 S. Karger AG, Basel

Fax +41 61 306 12 34
E-Mail karger@karger.ch
www.karger.com

The Journal Home Page is available at:
www.karger.com/aha

Acta
Hæmatologica

Recent Advances in the Understanding of Iron Metabolism and Related Diseases

Dedicated to Professor Ernest Beutler

Guest Editor
A. Victor Hoffbrand, London

22 figures, 6 in color, and 10 tables, 2009

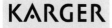 Basel · Freiburg · Paris · London · New York · Bangalore ·
Bangkok · Shanghai · Singapore · Tokyo · Sydney

S. Karger
Medical and Scientific Publishers
Basel • Freiburg • Paris • London •
New York • Bangalore • Bangkok •
Shanghai • Singapore • Tokyo • Sydney

Disclaimer
The statements, opinions and data contained in this publication are solely those of the individual authors and contributors
and not of the publisher and the editor(s). The appearance of
advertisements in the journal is not a warranty, endorsement,
or approval of the products or services advertised or of their
effectiveness, quality or safety. The publisher and the editor(s)
disclaim responsibility for any injury to persons or property
resulting from any ideas, methods, instructions or products
referred to in the content or advertisements.

Drug Dosage
The authors and the publisher have exerted every effort to ensure that drug selection and dosage set forth in this text are in
accord with current recommendations and practice at the time
of publication. However, in view of ongoing research, changes
in government regulations, and the constant flow of information relating to drug therapy and drug reactions, the reader is
urged to check the package insert for each drug for any change
in indications and dosage and for added warnings and precau-
tions. This is particularly important when the recommended
agent is a new and/or infrequently employed drug.

© Copyright 2009 by S. Karger AG,
P.O. Box, CH–4009 Basel (Switzerland)
Printed in Switzerland
on acid-free and non-aging paper (ISO 9706) by
Reinhardt Druck, Basel
ISBN 978–3–8055–9312–0
e-ISBN 978–3–8055–9313–7

KARGER

Fax +41 61 306 12 34
E-Mail karger@karger.ch
www.karger.com

Vol. 122, No. 2–3, 2009

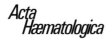

Contents

KARGER

Fax +41 61 306 12 34
E-Mail karger@karger.ch
www.karger.com

© 2009 S. Karger AG, Basel

Access to full text and tables of contents,
including tentative ones for forthcoming issues:
www.karger.com/aha_issues

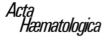
Acta Haematologica

Acta Haematol 2009;122:75–77
DOI: 10.1159/000243790

Published online: November 10, 2009

Recent Advances in the Understanding of Iron Metabolism and Iron-Related Diseases

A.V. Hoffbrand

Royal Free Hospital, London, UK

This special issue of *Acta Haematologica* brings together as authors many of the clinical scientists who have made major contributions to our understanding of iron metabolism and the mechanisms and treatment of iron-related diseases. It is dedicated to the memory of Prof. Ernest Beutler (1928–2008) who performed outstanding basic and clinical research on iron, as well as in many other areas of medicine (fig. 1).

My own interest in iron metabolism and iron overload began 40 years ago when I was at the Hammersmith Hospital in the Department of Haematology directed by Sir John Dacie. Two brothers with congenital sideroblastic anaemia were under my care. The younger boy needed regular blood transfusions and became iron overloaded. It was his need for effective iron chelation therapy that stimulated studies showing the efficacy of iron removal by subcutaneous desferrioxamine [1]. Pioneered in the USA by Propper et al. [2], this soon became standard chelation therapy for transfusional iron overload. It was shown to improve liver and cardiac function and overall survival in thalassaemia major. Many patients worldwide were still dying, however, from iron overload because the drug was too expensive in poor countries or because patients failed to comply with self-administered infusions on 5 or more days a week. Also, some apparently compliant patients were still developing an iron-induced cardiomyopathy which was difficult to predict from standard measures of body iron, such as serum ferritin or liver

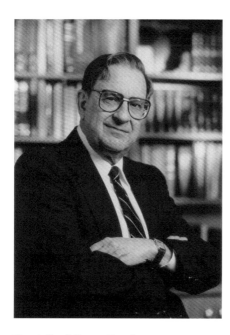

Fig. 1. Prof. Ernest Beutler.

iron. There remained an urgent need for a cheap, orally active iron chelator and for a non-invasive method of measuring cardiac iron.

The first report of an effective orally active iron chelator, deferiprone, appeared in 1987 [3] and this drug is still

Prof. A.V. Hoffbrand
Royal Free Hospital
Pond Street, London, NW3 2QG (UK)
Tel. +44 207 794 0500, ext. 33 258, Fax +44 207 431 4537
E-Mail v.hoffbrand@medsch.ucl.ac.uk

widely used. It appears to be particularly effective at removing cardiac iron. The development of the T2* MRI technique in Prof. Dudley Pennell's Department at the Royal Brompton Hospital in London fulfilled the need for a non-invasive reproducible technique for measuring cardiac iron [4]. It has enabled direct comparison of the efficacy of chelators on cardiac iron and prompted increased chelation for those patients with excess cardiac iron that would not otherwise have been detected [5].

A second orally active chelator, deferasirox, has subsequently been introduced with the advantage of once rather than three times daily administration and appears to be well tolerated [6]. The oral chelators used alone or in combination with desferrioxamine [7] have not only improved survival for thalassaemia major [8] but also made practical, iron chelation therapy for a wide range of other transfusion-dependent refractory anaemias.

Iron deficiency remains the most common anaemia in every country of the world with recent evidence that *Helicobacter pylori* and atrophic gastritis are common in its aetiology [9]. Simultaneously with these major clinical developments there has been a remarkable increase in the understanding of iron absorption, metabolism and cellular homeostasis by the discovery of a wide range of proteins involved in these processes [10, 11]. Ernest Beutler's laboratory contributed substantially to this new knowledge [12] and his investigations on genetic haemochromatosis have been critical in understanding genotypic/phenotypic relations in this disease [13]. Research into rare genetic diseases of iron overload and metabolism has helped to identify the proteins involved and elucidate their function [14, 15]. It has also revealed 'new' diseases such as iron-refractory iron deficiency anaemia [16] and different types of hereditary sideroblastic anaemias [17, 18], and improved our understanding and management of the more common anaemias of chronic inflammation, malignancy and heart failure reviewed in this issue by Agarwal and Prchal and by Silverberg and colleagues.

I first met Ernest Beutler in December 1967 in Toronto (Canada) at the coldest of ASH meetings. His outstanding research in enzyme deficiencies which cause haemolytic anaemia paralleled research of John Dacie at the Hammersmith Hospital. I reestablished contact with him in 1979 when he was President of the ASH meeting in the much warmer climate of Phoenix (Ariz., USA), when I was one of only five British haematologists attending. Since then he remained an intellectually stimulating, helpful and gracious friend to me, as to many other colleagues throughout the world. In 2003, he asked me to take part in an ASH Educational Symposium, despite my

advocacy of deferiprone, at a time when this was regarded, in the USA at least, as heretical. When I was first asked last year to edit an 'iron' issue for *Acta Haematologica*, I immediately invited Ernest Beutler to co-edit this with me. He declined because of illness but following his recent major research in establishing the role of matriptase-2 in iron metabolism, I invited him to write on this new topic. Five days before he died, he had the courtesy to suggest his colleague Dr. Pauline Lee might author this article in his place.

Ernest Beutler had a remarkable ability to achieve original, significant research in a wide range of topics, both at the clinical and basic science level. He made great contributions to our understanding of the genetic mechanisms of X-chromosome inactivation, glucose-6-phosphate dehydrogenase deficiency [19], other hereditary haemolytic anaemias, Tay-Sachs and Gaucher's disease [20], galactosaemia, iron metabolism and iron overload. He combined original scientific research in these and other topics with pioneering clinical research in the fields of haemochromatosis, bone marrow transplantation, the treatment of Gaucher's disease, blood storage, platelet transfusions and the use of new drugs such as chlorodoxyadenosine. In 1983, he introduced the first commercial bibliographic management software package, having written the programme himself. As well as over 800 original scientific papers, he authored 19 books and over 300 chapters. He was a truly outstanding haematologist, recognised by many awards and prizes. In 2007 he was the first recipient of the Wallace H. Coulter Award for Lifetime Achievement in Haematology. His career and the impact of his research on all haematologists have been more fully described by his son, Bruce Beutler [21]. We all miss his incisive intellect, originality, great sense of humour and warm friendship.

References

1 Hussain MA, Green N, Flynn DM, Hussein S, Hoffbrand AV: Subcutaneous infusion and intramuscular injection of desferrioxamine in patients with transfusional iron overload. Lancet 1976;ii:1278–1280.

2 Propper RD, Cooper B, Rufo RR, Nienhuis AW, Anderson WF, Bunn HF, Rosenthal A, Nathan DG: Continuous subcutaneous administration of desferrioxamine in patients with iron overload. N Engl J Med 1977;297:418–423.

3 Kontoghiorghes GJ, Aldouri M, Sheppard L, Hoffbrand AV: 1,2-Dimethyl-3-hydroxypyrid-4-one, an orally active chelator for treatment of iron overload. Lancet 1987;i:1294–1295.

4 Anderson LJ, Holden S, Davis B, Prescott E, Charrier CC, Bunce NH, Firmin DN, Wonke B, Porter J, Walker JM, Pennell DJ: Cardiovascular T2-star (T2*) magnetic resonance for the early diagnosis of myocardial iron overload. Eur Heart J 2001;22:2171–2179.

5 Anderson LJ, Westwood MA, Prescott E, Walker JM, Pennell DJ, Wonke B: Development of thalassemic iron overload cardiomyopathy despite low liver iron levels and meticulous compliance to desferrioxamine. Acta Haematol 2006;115:106–108.

6 Galanello R, Piga A, Alberti D, Rouan MC, Bigler H, Séchaud R: Safety, tolerability, and pharmacokinetics of ICL670, a new orally active iron-chelating agent in patients with transfusion-dependent iron overload due to β-thalassemia. J Clin Pharmacol 2003;43:565–572.

7 Wonke B, Wright S, Hoffbrand AV: Combined therapy with deferiprone and desferrioxamine. Br J Haematol 1998;103:361–364.

8 Modell B, Khan M, Darlison M, Westwood MA, Ingram D, Pennell DJ: Improved survival of thalassaemia major in the UK and relation to T2* cardiovascular magnetic resonance. J Cardiovasc Magn Reson 2008;10:42.

9 Hershko C, Hoffbrand AV, Keret D, Souroujon M, Maschler I, Monselise Y, Lahad A: Role of autoimmune gastritis, *Helicobacter pylori* and celiac disease in refractory or unexplained iron deficiency anemia. Haematologica 2005;90:585–595.

10 Nemeth E, Tuttle MS, Powelson J, Vaughn MB, Donovan A, Ward DM, Ganz T, Kaplan J: Hepcidin regulates cellular iron efflux by binding to ferroportin and inducing its internalization. Science 2004;306:2090–2093.

11 Lee PL, Beutler E: Regulation of hepcidin and iron-overload disease. Annu Rev Pathol 2009;4:489–515.

12 Du X, She E, Gelbart T, Truksa J, Lee P, Xia Y, Khovananth K, Mudd S, Mann N, Moresco EM, Beutler E, Beutler B: The serine protease TMPRSS6 is required to sense iron deficiency. Science 2008;320:1088–1092.

13 Beutler E, Felitti VJ, Koziol JA, Ho NJ, Gelbart T: Penetrance of 845G→A (C282Y) HFE hereditary haemochromatosis mutation in the USA. Lancet 2002;359:211–218.

14 Camaschella C: Understanding iron homeostasis through genetic analysis of hemochromatosis and related disorders. Blood 2005;106:3710–3717.

15 Zhang AS, Enns CA: Iron homeostasis: recently identified proteins provide insight into novel control mechanisms. J Biol Chem 2009;284:711–715.

16 Iolascon A, De Falco L, Beaumont C: Molecular basis of inherited microcytic anemia due to defects in iron acquisition or heme synthesis. Haematologica 2009;94:395–408.

17 Camaschella C: Recent advances in the understanding of inherited sideroblastic anaemia. Br J Haematol 2008;143:27–38.

18 Napier I, Ponka P, Richardson DR: Iron trafficking in the mitochondrion: novel pathways revealed by disease. Blood 2005;105:1867–1874.

19 Beutler E, Dern RJ, Alving AS: The hemolytic effect of primaquine. III. A study of primaquine-sensitive erythrocytes. J Lab Clin Med 1954;44:177–184.

20 Beutler E: Gaucher disease. Adv Genet 1995;32:17–49.

21 Beutler B: Obituary: Ernest Beutler (1928–2008). Haematologica 2009;94:154–156.

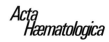

Acta Haematol 2009;122:78–86
DOI: 10.1159/000243791

Published online: November 10, 2009

The Role of Hepcidin in Iron Metabolism

Elizabeta Nemeth   Tomas Ganz

David Geffen School of Medicine, University of California, Los Angeles, Calif., USA

Key Words

Anemia of inflammation · Bone morphogenetic protein · Hemochromatosis · Hepcidin · Iron-loading anemia

Abstract

Hepcidin is the central regulator of systemic iron homeostasis. Dysregulation of hepcidin production results in a variety of iron disorders. Hepcidin deficiency is the cause of iron overload in hereditary hemochromatosis, iron-loading anemias, and hepatitis C. Hepcidin excess is associated with anemia of inflammation, chronic kidney disease and iron-refractory iron deficiency anemia. Diagnostic and therapeutic applications of this new knowledge are beginning to emerge. Dr. Ernest Beutler played a significant role in advancing our understanding of the function of hepcidin. This review is dedicated to his memory.

Copyright © 2009 S. Karger AG, Basel

Introduction

This review is dedicated to the memory of Dr. Ernest Beutler who had a career-long interest in iron homeostasis and its relationship to erythropoiesis. Guided by his legendary knowledge of all aspects of hematology and careful analysis of experimental and clinical data, he contributed much to modern hematology and was not afraid to challenge established beliefs. Even after he fell termi-

nally ill, he continued to make major contributions to the study of iron regulation. His ideas, attitudes, and achievements inspired us all.

Hepcidin Synthesis and Catabolism

The hormone hepcidin, a 25-amino-acid (aa) peptide, is the principal regulator of iron absorption and its distribution to tissues. Hepcidin is synthesized predominantly in hepatocytes, but its low levels of expression in other cells and tissues, including macrophages, adipocytes and brain, may also be important for the autocrine and paracrine control of iron fluxes at the local level.

Hepcidin is encoded as an 84-aa prepropeptide, containing an N-terminal 24-aa endoplasmic reticulum-targeting signal sequence. The 60-aa prohormone contains a consensus furin cleavage motif, and several proprotein convertases were reported to process hepcidin in vitro including furin, PACE4, PC5/6 and PC7/LPC. The processing step occurs in the Golgi apparatus, does not appear to be regulated, and only the mature peptide, but not the prohepcidin, was shown to be secreted from cells [1].

The mature hormone circulates in plasma and its binding to α_2-macroglobulin has been reported [2]. While this interaction was shown to promote hepcidin activity in vitro, the effect on hepcidin clearance is still unknown. A major route of hepcidin clearance is renal excretion. When kidney function is normal, urinary hepcidin con-

KARGER

Fax +41 61 306 12 34
E-Mail karger@karger.ch
www.karger.com

© 2009 S. Karger AG, Basel

Accessible online at:
www.karger.com/aha

Elizabeta Nemeth
Department of Medicine, UCLA
10833 LeConte Avenue, CHS 37-131
Los Angeles, CA 90095 (USA)
Tel. +1 310 825 7499, Fax +1 310 206 8766, E-Mail enemeth@mednet.ucla.edu

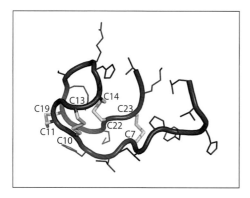

Fig. 1. Hepcidin structure with revised disulfide connectivities.

centrations correlate well with circulating hepcidin levels, with no apparent regulation of the excretion process. However, based on the comparison between serum and urinary concentrations, it appears that only 5% of hepcidin from plasma filtered in the kidneys ends up intact in the urine [3], suggesting that hepcidin may not be freely filtered in the glomerulus and/or that filtered hepcidin is reabsorbed and degraded in proximal tubules similarly to other small peptide hormones. Hepcidin may also be cleared by receptor-mediated endocytosis in tissues expressing its receptor ferroportin, as indicated by the accumulation of radiolabeled hepcidin in ferroportin-rich tissues [4] and the degradation of the endocytosed ferroportin-hepcidin complex in cultured cells. How much hepcidin catabolism occurs by renal clearance or by degradation in target tissues remains to be determined.

Hepcidin Structure

Structurally, the hepcidin peptide resembles a bent hairpin held together by four disulfide bonds. The disulfide connectivity was recently revised. NMR spectroscopy, partial reductive alkylation and Fourier transform mass spectroscopy were used to resolve ambiguities arising from the proximity of the four disulfides (Sasu et al., US patent application no. 2008/0213,277). The new model indicates that two bonds stabilize the antiparallel β-sheet, and two tether the bent conformation of the peptide (fig. 1). Our recent data indicate that hepcidin binding to its receptor requires the involvement of one of the disulfide bonds. However, considering that removal of individual bonds does not dramatically decrease hepcidin activity in vitro, multiple disulfide bonds must be capable of forming a contact with ferroportin.

The disulfide bonding pattern is strictly conserved across species that produce hepcidin – fish, amphibians, reptiles and mammals. Moreover, hepcidin from one species can bind to the receptor from an evolutionarily distant species, e.g. human and zebrafish hepcidin were active against mouse ferroportin [5]. Apart from the disulfide bonds, structure-function studies also revealed that the N-terminus of hepcidin is important for its iron-regulatory activity. The N-terminally truncated human 20-aa peptide was inactive both in vitro and in vivo indicating that this region may also contain contact residues for hepcidin interaction with its receptor.

The amphipathic structure of hepcidin and its extensive disulfide bonding are common characteristics of antimicrobial and antifungal peptides. However, hepcidin has only displayed modest antimicrobial properties in vitro at very high concentrations (10–30 μM), and the significance of its antimicrobial properties in vivo remains to be determined. Patients with hereditary hemochromatosis, a disease generally resulting from relative hepcidin deficiency, are reported to develop infections caused by unusual microorganisms (*Vibrio*, *Yersinia* and *Listeria*), but this susceptibility could be related to the bacteria benefitting from increased iron levels rather than from the loss of any direct antibacterial effect of hepcidin.

Iron-Regulatory Activity of Hepcidin

Hepcidin is the main regulator of plasma iron concentrations. Injection of hepcidin into mice resulted in a dramatic drop in serum iron within just 1 h [4]. Even though hepcidin is rapidly cleared from the plasma, the effect of a single dose was apparent for up to 72 h, likely because of the time required to resynthesize sufficient amounts of the hepcidin receptor, ferroportin.

Chronic overexpression of hepcidin causes iron-restricted anemia in mice and humans, typically manifested as microcytic, hypochromic anemia. Conversely, hepcidin deficiency in mice and humans results in iron overload with iron deposition in the liver and other parenchyma, and sparing of the macrophage-rich spleen. Complete absence of hepcidin in humans causes juvenile hemochromatosis, the most severe form of hereditary hemochromatosis.

The phenotypes of hepcidin excess and deficiency indicate that hepcidin inhibits intestinal iron uptake and the release of iron from macrophages recycling old red blood cells (fig. 2). When hepcidin was overexpressed during embryonic development, fetuses developed severe

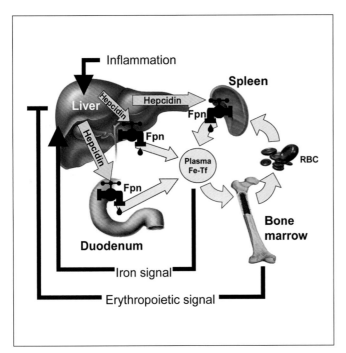

Fig. 2. Hepcidin-ferroportin (Fpn) interaction determines the flow of iron into plasma. Hepcidin concentration is in turn regulated by iron, erythropoietic activity and inflammation.

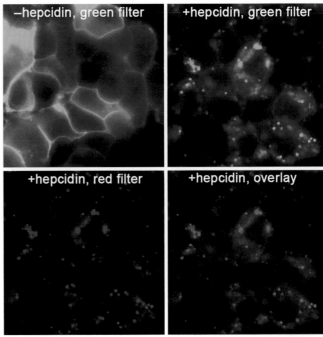

Fig. 3. Hepcidin binding to ferroportin causes internalization of the receptor-ligand complex, and their eventual degradation. HEK293 cells expressing ferroportin-GFP were treated with Texas-red-labeled hepcidin and imaged using fluorescent microscopy.

iron deficiency anemia and most died at birth indicating that hepcidin also inhibited the placental transport of iron [6]. Hepcidin also appears to block, at least partially, the export of stored iron from hepatocytes as indicated by hepatic iron accumulation in mice carrying hepcidin-overproducing tumors.

Hepcidin derived from extrahepatic sources may also exert control over local iron fluxes within tissues in which hepcidin is produced. For example, the central nervous system is separated from the plasma by the blood-brain barrier, and circulating hepcidin may not be transported across this barrier. However, brain tissue itself was reported to express hepcidin, allowing the possibility of iron regulation independent of the systemic control.

Mechanism of Hepcidin Action

Hepcidin acts by modulating cellular iron export through ferroportin to plasma and extracellular fluid (fig. 2). Ferroportin is both the hepcidin receptor and the only known cellular iron exporter in vertebrates. Ferroportin is expressed on cells that act as professional iron handlers in the body: duodenal enterocytes absorbing dietary iron, macrophages in liver and spleen recycling old erythrocytes, hepatocytes storing iron and placental trophoblasts transferring iron to the fetus during pregnancy [7]. Ferroportin is also expressed in erythroid precursor cells, and it has been proposed that its presence enhances the sensitivity of precursors to systemic iron levels and helps determine their commitment to expansion and differentiation [8]. The complete loss of ferroportin expression in zebrafish and mouse models was shown to be embryonic lethal due to the inability of embryonic trophoblasts to transfer iron from the mother to the embryo. In the selective ferroportin knockout mice that preserved placental ferroportin, the newborn mice lacking ferroportin developed severe iron deficiency anemia due to low dietary iron absorption, and defective release of iron from hepatic storage and iron-recycling macrophages [7].

Posttranslational control of ferroportin levels by its ligand hepcidin is the major mode of ferroportin regulation. The binding of hepcidin to ferroportin triggers the internalization and degradation of the receptor-ligand complex [9] (fig. 3). The binding likely involves disulfide exchange between one of disulfide bonds of hepcidin and the exofacial ferroportin thiol residue Cys326. Patients with C326S mutations develop early-onset iron overload, and the mutant ferroportin lost its ability to bind hepcidin in vitro [10]. Once internalized, the hepcidin-ferroportin complex is degraded in lysosomes and cellular iron export ceases.

Ferroportin expression can also be regulated independently of hepcidin, by cellular iron content. Cellular iron has been shown to have an effect both at the transcriptional and translational level, the latter through a mechanism involving cytoplasmic iron-regulatory proteins and their corresponding binding sites in the 5′-region of one of the ferroportin mRNA isoforms [8].

Interestingly, the mechanism of iron transport by ferroportin has remained unexplored, and is one of the important challenges in advancing our understanding of cellular and systemic iron regulation.

Regulation of Hepcidin

Hepcidin is homeostatically regulated by iron and erythropoietic activity. Iron excess stimulates hepcidin production, and increased concentrations of the hormone in turn block dietary iron absorption thus preventing further iron loading (fig. 2). Conversely, hepcidin is suppressed in iron deficiency, allowing increased absorption of dietary iron and replenishment of iron stores. Increased erythropoietic activity also suppresses hepcidin production. Apart from enhancing iron absorption, this enables the rapid release of stored iron from macrophages and hepatocytes and augments the supply of iron for erythropoiesis. The molecular mechanisms underlying hepcidin regulation by iron and erythropoiesis are areas of intense investigation but are still incompletely understood. Hepcidin is also increased in inflammation and infection, and it is presumed that this regulation evolved as a host defense strategy to limit iron availability to microorganisms.

Hepcidin Regulation by Iron

Hepcidin is likely regulated by both circulating iron transferrin (Tf) and intracellular iron stores. Although the iron-sensing molecules for extracellular versus intracellular iron seem to be different, they both appear to utilize the bone morphogenetic protein (BMP) pathway to alter hepcidin expression. The BMP pathway has emerged as the critical regulator of hepcidin expression. BMPs control a variety of biological processes during embryonic and postnatal development, and signal by bind-

ing to several types of BMP receptors. This results in phosphorylation of cytoplasmic Smad1/Smad5/Smad8 which associate with the common mediator Smad4 and translocate into the nucleus where they act as transcription factors. Liver-specific disruption of Smad4 in mice resulted in iron overload due to severely decreased hepcidin expression [11]. Typically, BMP signaling is modulated by coreceptors, among which hemojuvelin (HJV) is specific for iron regulation. Humans with disruptive HJV mutations or HJV knockout mice have iron overload as severe as that caused by ablation of hepcidin, with no other apparent problems [12].

In addition to the BMP/HJV pathway, other factors are necessary for hepcidin regulation by iron Tf. These include Tf receptor 2 (TfR2) and HFE, two molecules which are mutated in the adult forms of hereditary hemochromatosis. TfR2 is a homolog of TfR1, the receptor essential for the uptake of iron Tf by erythrocytes, and also expressed on most other cell types. TfR2 is primarily expressed in the liver, and while its mRNA expression is not affected by iron levels, its iron-sensing function appears to involve the stabilization of TfR2 protein after binding of iron Tf [13]. HFE, a protein similar to MHC class I molecules, does not bind iron directly but instead interacts with iron-binding proteins, TfR1 and TfR2. It has been proposed that HFE shuttles between TfR1 and TfR2 depending on iron Tf concentrations [14]. In the absence of iron Tf, HFE associates with TfR1, but when iron Tf binds to TfR1, HFE is displaced and associates with TfR2 instead. Gao et al. [15] recently demonstrated that interaction of HFE and TfR2 is required for hepcidin induction in response to iron Tf. How the HFE/TfR2 complex signals to the hepcidin promoter is still unclear, but it appears to involve the BMP pathway. Inhibitors of BMP signaling (noggin and sHJV) prevented hepcidin mRNA increase after holo-Tf treatment in primary hepatocytes in vitro [16]. Because HFE and TfR2 were reported to interact with HJV, it is possible that binding of iron Tf to TfR1 and TfR2 initiates the formation of a supercomplex composed of HFE, TfR2, HJV and BMP receptors (fig. 4).

Apart from iron Tf, hepcidin may also be regulated by iron stores, presumably by some form of intracellular iron. HFE and TfR2 are not required for this regulation as mice and humans with HFE and TfR2 mutations are still capable of decreasing hepcidin levels after iron depletion. Although the mechanism of intracellular iron sensing is unclear, new evidence suggests that it may center on BMP6 [17]. First, BMP6 mRNA expression was shown to be regulated by iron loading: mice fed for 3 weeks with low-iron (<3 ppm) or high-iron (8,300 ppm)

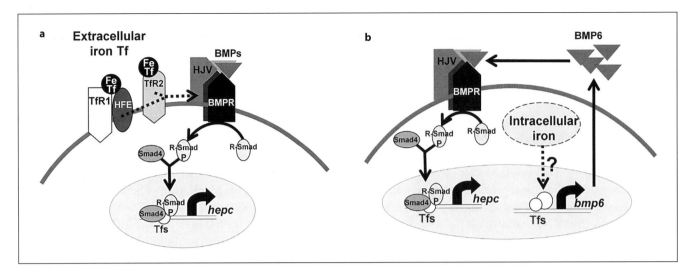

Fig. 4. A model of hepcidin regulation by iron Tf (**a**) and intracellular iron (**b**). **a** Increased iron Tf concentrations stabilize TfR2 protein, HFE is displaced from TfR1 and associates with TfR2. The HFE-TfR2 complex likely interacts with the HJV-BMP receptor (BMPR), BMP signaling is potentiated and hepcidin transcription increases. **b** Elevated intracellular iron increases BMP6 production. Secreted BMP6 binds to the HJV-BMPR complex, stimulates Smad signaling, and increases hepcidin transcription.

diet had lower and higher BMP6 mRNA, respectively, than mice fed an iron-balanced diet (200 ppm). Moreover, BMP6 protein was shown to interact directly and specifically with the coreceptor HJV. Finally, the disruption of BMP6 in mice resulted in very low expression of hepcidin and severe iron overload, but no other significant abnormalities. While these studies highlight the specific role of BMP6 in hepcidin regulation, it remains to be determined how the production of BMP6 itself is regulated by iron.

Additional molecules were shown to interact with HJV and modify its cell surface expression, including a protease (TMPRSS6) and a large multifunctional transmembrane protein (neogenin), but whether these processes are regulated by iron or other signals remains to be determined.

Hepcidin Regulation by Erythropoietic Activity

Hepcidin is decreased in iron deficiency anemia, hemolytic anemia, and anemias with ineffective erythropoiesis. The mechanisms mediating hepcidin suppression in these conditions, however, may not be the same. While the molecular details of the pathways involved are unclear, they may include soluble protein(s) produced by the developing erythroblasts in the bone marrow, decreased circulating or stored iron, and hypoxia.

In mouse models of anemias caused by bleeding or hemolysis, two studies showed that hepcidin suppression was dependent on intact erythropoietic activity. When erythropoiesis was inhibited using cytotoxic agents or irradiation, hepcidin mRNA did not decrease despite severe anemia [18].

Two proteins produced by erythroid precursors, growth differentiation factor 15 (GDF15) and twisted gastrulation protein (TWSG1), have been proposed to mediate hepcidin suppression in anemias with ineffective erythropoiesis [19]. GDF15 is a member of the TGF-β superfamily, and although GDF15 knockout or transgenic mice do not have obvious iron abnormalities, larger doses of GDF15 do suppress hepcidin mRNA in vitro. Such doses are comparable to the levels of GDF15 observed in β-thalassemia and congenital dyserythropoietic anemia type I, diseases with massive overproduction of GDF15.

TWSG1 is a BMP-binding protein produced early during erythroblast maturation. TWSG1 also suppresses hepcidin in vitro, and it acts by interfering with BMP-dependent hepcidin regulation. Not much is known about TWSG1 expression in humans, but TWSG1 expression was increased in a mouse model of thalassemia.

Hepcidin is decreased by hypoxia, but the physiological relevance of this regulation is still uncertain. Alterations in the hypoxia-inducible factor (HIF) pathway in vivo can affect hepcidin expression. Liver-specific stabilization of HIF in mice, achieved by disruption of von Hippel-Lindau (VHL), resulted in markedly decreased hepcidin mRNA levels [20]. When these mice had an additional gene knocked out encoding a component of the HIF transcriptional complex, hepcidin levels were not suppressed any more. Whether HIF directly regulates hepcidin transcription is still unresolved. One study showed that HIF-1 bound to the mouse and human hepcidin promoters, but another study found that overexpression or knockdown of HIF-1 did not alter hepcidin expression in HepG2 cells. The indirect effects of hypoxia may be more important. Hypoxia-induced erythropoietin (EPO) could act as an intermediate and suppress hepcidin production through EPO-stimulated proliferation of erythroblasts, secreted products of erythrocyte precursors, and eventually increased iron utilization for hemoglobin synthesis.

Hepcidin Regulation by Inflammation

Hepcidin synthesis is rapidly increased by infection and inflammation. Of the specific pathways, IL-6 was shown to be a prominent inducer of hepcidin, through a STAT3-dependent transcriptional mechanism. In human volunteers infused with IL-6, urinary hepcidin excretion was increased several fold within 2 h after infusion [21]. In mice, other cytokines can also directly regulate hepcidin production, since IL-6 knockout mice with chronic inflammation had elevated hepcidin mRNA similarly to wild-type mice. IL-1 was shown to increase hepcidin mRNA in mouse hepatocytes independently of IL-6, but it remains to be determined whether there are any species-specific differences in hepcidin regulation by inflammation.

Hepcidin and Diseases

Inappropriate production of hepcidin contributes to the pathogenesis of various iron disorders (table 1). Relative deficiency in hepcidin is associated with development of iron overload, whereas relative excess of hepcidin causes iron restriction and anemia.

Diseases of Hepcidin Deficiency

Hepcidin deficiency results in the development of systemic iron overload because of excessive iron absorption. In the absence of hepcidin, ferroportin concentrations on the basolateral surface of enterocytes are increased, leading to enhanced transport of dietary iron into plasma. In hepcidin deficiency, macrophages also display increased ferroportin on their cell membranes and thus export more iron. Excess plasma iron accumulates in organs in which iron uptake exceeds the rate of iron export. The

Table 1. Iron disorders associated with inappropriate hepcidin production

Defect in hepcidin production	Disease
Hepcidin deficiency	hereditary hemochromatosis iron-loading anemias hepatitis C
Hepcidin excess	anemia of inflammation chronic kidney diseases iron-refractory iron deficiency anemia

liver is most commonly affected by iron overload due to the avid uptake of non-Tf-bound iron by hepatocytes. Iron overload of other organs appears to correlate broadly with the rate of iron absorption. Rapid accumulation of iron, such as seen with severe hepcidin deficiency (juvenile hemochromatosis or thalassemia intermedia), is associated with prominent deposition of iron in the heart and some endocrine organs. Although hepcidin deficiency is the common denominator of several different iron overload disorders, the molecular mechanisms that cause hepcidin deficiency are diverse.

In hereditary hemochromatosis [reviewed by Camaschella and Poggiali in this issue; pp 140–145], hepcidin deficiency results either from mutations in the hepcidin gene itself, or in the genes encoding hepcidin regulators. A very rare form of hemochromatosis is not associated with hepcidin deficiency, but with ferroportin resistance to hepcidin. Hepcidin regulators which are mutated in hereditary hemochromatosis include HFE, TfR2 and HJV, the molecules involved in sensing of iron and subsequent signal transduction. Importantly, the degree of hepcidin deficiency correlates with the severity of iron overload, so that the most severe form of hemochromatosis, juvenile hemochromatosis, develops with mutations in the hepcidin or HJV genes, where hepcidin levels are completely or nearly absent. TfR2 and HFE mutations result in a milder phenotype, particularly HFE mutations, which have a lower clinical penetrance.

Phlebotomy is currently the main treatment for patients with hereditary hemochromatosis. Although this is effective at removing excess iron, complete iron depletion appears to result in a further decrease in hepcidin levels which would be expected to enhance dietary iron absorption and increase the need for phlebotomy. Further studies are needed to establish whether less iron depletion, which would not lower hepcidin levels as much, would still be safe for patients and allow less frequent phlebotomy.

In iron-loading anemias, such as β-thalassemia and congenital dyserythropoietic anemias, urinary and serum hepcidin are severely decreased despite systemic iron overload [22]. The signal causing hepcidin suppression appears to be generated by high erythropoietic activity and outweighs the effects of iron overload on hepcidin regulation. As mentioned earlier, GDF15 and TWSG1 are two erythroid-produced factors that may contribute to hepcidin suppression in these syndromes. Transfusions increase hepcidin levels, presumably due to both the alleviation of ineffective erythropoiesis and increased iron load. Interestingly, patients with thalassemia intermedia were shown to have liver iron concentrations similar to those of regularly transfused thalassemia major patients, but because of the different hepcidin levels, the cellular distribution of iron in the liver was different. In thalassemia intermedia, similar to hereditary hemochromatosis, iron was heavily deposited in hepatocytes, whereas higher hepcidin levels in thalassemia major caused a shift of iron into macrophages. It is therefore possible that therapeutic hepcidin could be useful in thalassemia to shift the iron from the parenchyma to macrophages, where it is less toxic.

Hepcidin levels were also reported to be low in patients with chronic hepatitis C, a disease frequently accompanied by hepatic iron overload, which worsens liver damage. The mechanism by which hepatitis C virus suppresses hepcidin synthesis is not well understood, but was reported to include the virus-induced oxidative stress.

Diseases of Hepcidin Excess

Human syndromes of hepcidin overproduction suggest, and mouse models demonstrate, that elevated hepcidin is sufficient to cause hypoferremia and anemia [23]. Mice administered a single intraperitoneal injection of synthetic hepcidin developed hypoferremia within 1 h which lasted for almost 3 days [4]. Transgenic mice strongly overexpressing hepcidin during embryonic development developed severe microcytic, hypochromic anemia in utero [6], and weaker hepcidin overexpression caused mild-to-moderate anemia which was associated with iron-restricted erythropoiesis [23]. The phenotype develops from hepcidin-mediated inhibition of iron recycling and absorption. Decreased flow of iron into plasma results in hypoferremia, and because most of the iron in plasma is destined for the bone marrow, lower iron availability affects hemoglobin synthesis and erythrocyte production. In human disease, elevated hepcidin may

contribute to anemia observed in inflammatory disorders, chronic kidney disease (CKD), hepcidin-producing hepatic adenomas and hereditary iron-refractory iron deficiency anemia (IRIDA).

In inflammatory disorders, hepcidin production is stimulated by increased cytokines, prominently including IL-6. Chronic hepcidin-mediated iron restriction would be expected to eventually lead to anemia of inflammation (AI) [for further information, see the review by Agarwal and Prchal in this issue; pp 103–108]. Elevated hepcidin was observed in rheumatologic diseases, inflammatory bowel disease, multiple myeloma, and critical illness, but whether hepcidin is a necessary factor in the pathogenesis of anemia in each of these disorders has not yet been established with certainty. Studies in mice moderately overexpressing hepcidin indicate that increased hepcidin not only causes iron restriction but also blunted erythropoietic response to EPO, characteristic of AI. Hepcidin does not appear to decrease red blood cell survival, another feature associated with AI. The role of hepcidin in the suppression of EPO, sometimes seen in AI, is unclear. Studies of interventions that selectively reduce hepcidin will be necessary to determine how essential the role of hepcidin is in inflammation-induced anemia.

Hepcidin concentrations were reported to be increased in CKD patients [for further information, see the review by Silverberg et al. in this issue; pp 109–119]. This could be caused by inflammation which frequently accompanies CKD, but even patients without significant inflammation had elevated hepcidin levels which progressively increased with the severity of CKD. Because hepcidin is cleared, at least in part, by filtration in the kidney, decreased kidney function is the likely factor contributing to this phenomenon. Indeed, some studies reported an inverse correlation between glomerular filtration rate and serum hepcidin. It has been postulated that high hepcidin may be the reason for EPO resistance commonly observed in CKD patients. Two initial studies, however, reported no correlation between hepcidin-25 levels and EPO dose, raising questions about the usefulness of hepcidin as a predictor of patients' response to EPO. However, the ability of high EPO doses to suppress hepcidin synthesis may confound these studies.

IRIDA is a disease characterized by congenital hypochromic, microcytic anemia, refractory to treatment with oral iron, and only partially responsive to parenteral iron. The phenotype has been described almost 30 years ago, but its molecular basis has only recently been unraveled. IRIDA is caused by increased hepcidin production due to mutations in the hepcidin suppressor, TMPRSS6. The mechanisms are covered in more detail in the review by Lee [this issue; pp 87–96].

Clinical Applications of Hepcidin

Diagnostics

Considering that hepcidin is fundamentally involved in the pathogenesis of many iron disorders, measurements of hepcidin concentrations in biological fluids would be expected to facilitate the diagnosis of those diseases (table 1). The evaluation of the diagnostic potential of hepcidin has only recently become possible with the development of assays for bioactive mature hepcidin in serum and urine. The methodologies include competitive ELISAs using biotinylated or radioiodinated hepcidin as tracers, and several mass-spectrometry-based assays (matrix-assisted laser desorption ionization/time of flight/mass spectrometry, surface-enhanced laser desorption/ionization, and liquid chromatography coupled with tandem mass spectrometric) using as internal standards isotopically labeled hepcidin or shorter hepcidin mutants. Measurements of prohepcidin in serum have also been reported, but these did not correlate with mature hepcidin concentrations indicating that prohepcidin is inadequate as a substitute for measuring biologically relevant hepcidin.

Although promising, the utility of hepcidin for the diagnosis and prognosis of iron disorders needs to be evaluated in larger clinical studies.

Therapeutics

As most types of hereditary hemochromatosis are caused by hepcidin deficiency, hepcidin agonists should be useful for the prevention or treatment of these diseases. The proof of principle was demonstrated when iron overload was successfully prevented in HFE knockout mice made to transgenically express hepcidin [24]. In practice, however, many patients are first diagnosed with advanced iron overload. In that scenario, hepcidin agonists may be useful as adjuncts to therapeutic phlebotomy, where they would act to redistribute iron to macrophages and away from parenchymal cells, block further iron absorption and eventually eliminate the need for maintenance phlebotomy. A similar approach may be useful in hepatitis C patients with hepatic iron overload.

In β-thalassemias and other iron-loading anemias, hepcidin agonists may help control intestinal iron absorption, which is the sole cause of iron overload in patients not receiving transfusions. Unlike in hereditary hemochromatosis, an important consideration in this disease is whether hepcidin administration would negatively affect erythropoiesis. For the patients with transfusion-related iron overload, the utility of hepcidin agonists is not clear. It is possible that hepcidin could alter the distribution of iron from parenchyma to macrophages where it is less harmful.

Hepcidin antagonists would be expected to benefit patients with diseases of hepcidin excess, manifested as iron-restricted anemia and, eventually, as systemic iron deficiency. This use of hepcidin antagonists was conceptually validated in a mouse model of AI induced by injections of Brucella abortus. While mice injected with EPO alone showed little response, combination therapy using EPO and hepcidin-neutralizing antibody or hepcidin siRNA restored normal hemoglobin levels (Sasu et al., US patent application no. 2008/0213,277). Apart from those directly interfering with hepcidin activity, other agents which target pathways regulating hepcidin production have also been described. Dorsomorphin, a small-molecule inhibitor of BMP signaling, prevented hepcidin induction by iron in vivo [25]. Soluble HJV, also acting as an antagonist of BMP signaling, decreased hepcidin baseline expression in mice and concurrently increased liver iron content. Finally, in patients with inflammatory diseases, anemia may be responsive to anti-cytokine therapies such as anti-IL-6 antibody. Undoubtedly, future studies will assess the risks and relative benefits of these treatment approaches.

Conclusions

Since the first reports of hepcidin almost a decade ago, our understanding of the function of hepcidin in iron homeostasis has expanded tremendously, a development that Dr. Ernest Beutler contributed to and greatly enjoyed. Diagnostic and therapeutic applications of the new knowledge are beginning to emerge. These advances will improve the health and well-being of the many millions of patients with iron disorders.

Acknowledgment

This study was supported by a grant from the National Institutes of Health (R01 DK082717).

References

1 Valore EV, Ganz T: Posttranslational processing of hepcidin in human hepatocytes is mediated by the prohormone convertase furin. Blood Cells Mol Dis 2008;40:132–138.

2 Peslova G, Petrak J, Kuzelova K, Hrdy I, Halada P, Kuchel PW, Soe-Lin S, Ponka P, Sutak R, Becker E, Huang ML, Suryo RY, Richardson DR, Vyoral D: Hepcidin, the hormone of iron metabolism, is bound specifically to alpha-2-macroglobulin in blood. Blood 2009;113:6225–6236.

3 Ganz T, Olbina G, Girelli D, Nemeth E, Westerman M: Immunoassay for human serum hepcidin. Blood 2008;112:4292–4297.

4 Rivera S, Nemeth E, Gabayan V, Lopez MA, Farshidi D, Ganz T: Synthetic hepcidin causes rapid dose-dependent hypoferremia and is concentrated in ferroportin-containing organs. Blood 2005;106:2196–2199.

5 Nemeth E, Preza GC, Jung CL, Kaplan J, Waring AJ, Ganz T: The N-terminus of hepcidin is essential for its interaction with ferroportin: structure-function study. Blood 2006;107:328–333.

6 Nicolas G, Bennoun M, Porteu A, Mativet S, Beaumont C, Grandchamp B, Sirito M, Sawadogo M, Kahn A, Vaulont S: Severe iron deficiency anemia in transgenic mice expressing liver hepcidin. Proc Natl Acad Sci USA 2002;99:4596–4601.

7 Donovan A, Lima CA, Pinkus JL, Pinkus GS, Zon LI, Robine S, Andrews NC: The iron exporter ferroportin/Slc40a1 is essential for iron homeostasis. Cell Metab 2005;1:191–200.

8 Zhang DL, Hughes RM, Ollivierre-Wilson H, Ghosh MC, Rouault TA: A ferroportin transcript that lacks an iron-responsive element enables duodenal and erythroid precursor cells to evade translational repression. Cell Metab 2009;9:461–473.

9 Nemeth E, Tuttle MS, Powelson J, Vaughn MB, Donovan A, Ward DM, Ganz T, Kaplan J: Hepcidin regulates cellular iron efflux by binding to ferroportin and inducing its internalization. Science 2004;306:2090–2093.

10 Fernandes A, Preza GC, Phung Y, De Domenico I, Kaplan J, Ganz T, Nemeth E: The molecular basis of hepcidin-resistant hereditary hemochromatosis. Blood 2009;114:437–443.

11 Wang RH, Li C, Xu X, Zheng Y, Xiao C, Zerfas P, Cooperman S, Eckhaus M, Rouault T, Mishra L, Deng CX: A role of SMAD4 in iron metabolism through the positive regulation of hepcidin expression. Cell Metab 2005;2:399–409.

12 Niederkofler V, Salie R, Arber S: Hemojuvelin is essential for dietary iron sensing, and its mutation leads to severe iron overload. J Clin Invest 2005;115:2180–2186.

13 Johnson MB, Chen J, Murchison N, Green FA, Enns CA: Transferrin receptor 2: evidence for ligand-induced stabilization and redirection to a recycling pathway. Mol Biol Cell 2007;18:743–754.

14 Goswami T, Andrews NC: Hereditary hemochromatosis protein, HFE, interaction with transferrin receptor 2 suggests a molecular mechanism for mammalian iron sensing. J Biol Chem 2006;281:28494–28498.

15 Gao J, Chen J, Kramer M, Tsukamoto H, Zhang AS, Enns CA: Interaction of the hereditary hemochromatosis protein HFE with transferrin receptor 2 is required for transferrin-induced hepcidin expression. Cell Metab 2009;9:217–227.

16 Lin L, Valore EV, Nemeth E, Goodnough JB, Gabayan V, Ganz T: Iron transferrin regulates hepcidin synthesis in primary hepatocyte culture through hemojuvelin and BMP2/4. Blood 2007;110:2182–2189.

17 Camaschella C: BMP6 orchestrates iron metabolism. Nat Genet 2009;41:386–388.

18 Pak M, Lopez MA, Gabayan V, Ganz T, Rivera S: Suppression of hepcidin during anemia requires erythropoietic activity. Blood 2006;108:3730–3735.

19 Tanno T, Bhanu NV, Oneal PA, Goh SH, Staker P, Lee YT, Moroney JW, Reed CH, Luban NL, Wang RH, Eling TE, Childs R, Ganz T, Leitman SF, Fucharoen S, Miller JL: High levels of GDF15 in thalassemia suppress expression of the iron regulatory protein hepcidin. Nat Med 2007;13:1096–1101.

20 Peyssonnaux C, Zinkernagel AS, Schuepbach RA, Rankin E, Vaulont S, Haase VH, Nizet V, Johnson RS: Regulation of iron homeostasis by the hypoxia-inducible transcription factors (HIFs). J Clin Invest 2007;117:1926–1932.

21 Nemeth E, Rivera S, Gabayan V, Keller C, Taudorf S, Pedersen BK, Ganz T: IL-6 mediates hypoferremia of inflammation by inducing the synthesis of the iron regulatory hormone hepcidin. J Clin Invest 2004;113:1271–1276.

22 Nemeth E, Ganz T: Hepcidin and iron-loading anemias. Haematologica 2006;91:727–732.

23 Roy CN, Mak HH, Akpan I, Losyev G, Zurakowski D, Andrews NC: Hepcidin antimicrobial peptide transgenic mice exhibit features of the anemia of inflammation. Blood 2007;109:4038–4044.

24 Nicolas G, Viatte L, Lou DQ, Bennoun M, Beaumont C, Kahn A, Andrews NC, Vaulont S: Constitutive hepcidin expression prevents iron overload in a mouse model of hemochromatosis. Nat Genet 2003;34:97–101.

25 Yu PB, Hong CC, Sachidanandan C, Babitt JL, Deng DY, Hoyng SA, Lin HY, Bloch KD, Peterson RT: Dorsomorphin inhibits BMP signals required for embryogenesis and iron metabolism. Nat Chem Biol 2008;4:33–41.

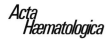

Acta Haematol 2009;122:87–96
DOI: 10.1159/000243792

Published online: November 10, 2009

Role of Matriptase-2 (TMPRSS6) in Iron Metabolism

Pauline Lee

Scripps Research Institute, La Jolla, Calif., USA

Key Words

CUB · Hemojuvelin · Hepcidin · Iron · LDLa · Matriptase ·
TMPRSS · Type II serine protease

Abstract

Iron, an essential element for life, is regulated primarily at the level of uptake, storage, and transport in order to maintain sufficient availability for normal physiology. The key protein in iron homeostasis is a 25-amino-acid peptide, hepcidin, which modulates the amount of iron in the circulation by binding and promoting the degradation of the iron exporter ferroportin. Given the central importance of hepcidin, recent studies have focused on how iron is sensed and how the iron signal is transmitted to hepcidin. Mutations in a type II serine protease, matriptase-2/TMPRSS6, were recently identified to be associated with severe iron deficiency caused by inappropriately high levels of hepcidin expression. A key biologically relevant substrate for the proteolytic activity of matriptase-2/TMPRSS6 was found to be hemojuvelin, a cell surface protein that regulates hepcidin expression through a BMP/SMAD pathway. In this review, we discuss the putative role of matriptase-2/TMPRSS6 in iron homeostasis.

Copyright © 2009 S. Karger AG, Basel

Introduction

Recent identification of the importance of TMPRSS6/matriptase-2 in iron homeostasis has resulted in the publication of several excellent review articles [1–3]. This review is written as a special tribute to Dr. Ernest Beutler, for whom the understanding of iron homeostasis was one of his many research passions. It will include work done in his laboratory the final year of his life and shortly afterwards, and will discuss some aspects of the field not covered by previous review articles.

Matriptase-2, also called TMPRSS6, is a type II plasma membrane serine protease (TTSP). The 811-amino-acid (aa) human protein is synthesized as an inactive zymogen and autoactivated by proteolytic cleavage. Structurally, matriptase-2 contains a short 54-aa N-terminal cytoplasmic domain, a membrane-spanning region, an SEA (sea urchin sperm protein, enteropeptidase, and agrin) domain, 2 CUB [Cls/Clr, urchin embryonic growth factor, and bone morphogeneic protein (BMP)-1] domains, three LDLa (low-density-lipoprotein receptor, class A) domains, and a trypsin-like serine protease domain containing the catalytic triad of histidine, aspartate, and serine residues (fig. 1). Matriptase-2 contains 38 conserved cysteine residues predicted to form 18 extracellular intramolecular disulfide bonds, three of which are within the catalytic protease domain (C593-C609, C724-C738, and C749-C778). One of the disulfide bonds (C559-C679)

KARGER

Fax +41 61 306 12 34
E-Mail karger@karger.ch
www.karger.com

© 2009 S. Karger AG, Basel

Accessible online at:
www.karger.com/aha

Pauline Lee, PhD
Department of Molecular and Experimental Medicine, Scripps Research Institute
10550 North Torrey Pines Road, MEM 215
La Jolla, CA 92037 (USA)
Tel. +1 858 784 2217, Fax +1 858 784 2083, E-Mail plee@scripps.edu

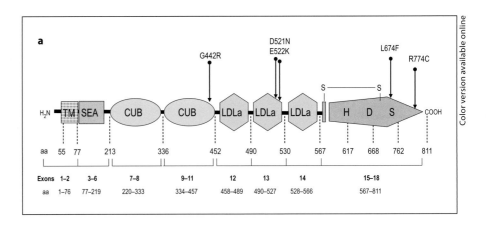

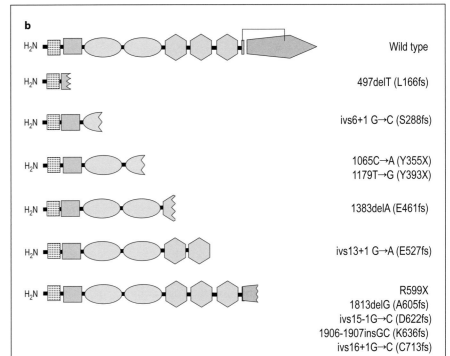

Fig. 1. Schematic model of matriptase-2. **a** Structurally, matriptase-2 contains a short N-terminal cytoplasmic domain, a membrane-spanning region (TM), an SEA domain, 2 CUB domains, three LDLa domains, and a trypsin-like serine protease domain with the highly conserved catalytic triad of histidine (H617), aspartic acid (D668), and serine (S762) residues. Coding region mutations resulting in an aa change that have been identified in IRIDA patients are indicated by arrows [17, 20, 30]. **b** Schematic model of matriptase-2 truncation mutants identified in IRIDA patients [17–20, 30].

serves to hold the protease domain to the stem region after proteolytic autoactivation. The unpaired cysteine residue in the SEA domain and the unpaired intracellular cysteine residue have the potential to participate in intermolecular bonding. Matriptase-2 lacks group A scavenger receptor domains representative of other members of the hepsin/TMPRSS subfamily and lacks frizzled domains present in the corin subfamily of TTSPs [1]. The differences in protein structure and differences in aa sequence homology between the TMPRSS and matriptase subfamilies suggest that TMPRSS6 is a misnomer and its designation as matriptase-2 is more accurate [1]. For this reason, for the remainder of this review, the protein will be referred to as matriptase-2, but the gene will be referred to as *TMPRSS6*.

SEA domains are *O*-glycosylated and may play a role in binding to other cell surface glycoproteins or substrate proteins. Within the SEA domains of several membrane proteins is a conserved cleavage site, GSVIV (enteropeptidase), GSVIA (matriptase), and GSVVV (mucin) by which proteolytic processing after the glycine residue sheds the protein from the cell surface. Matriptase-2, which has been reported to be shed from the cell surface [4], contains the motif GSLRV in the homologous region of the SEA domain that might be the putative cleavage site.

Table 1. Matriptase-2 protein and synthetic peptide substrates

Matriptase-2 cleavage of synthetic peptides		
Artificial	Boc QAR↓-Amc	[8]
Artificial	Boc QNR↓-Amc	[8]
Filaggrin	RKR↓R↓GSRG	[12]
Trask (CDCP1)	KQR↓SKFVP	[12]
$α_E β_7$ Integrin	RQRR↓ALEK	[12]
Matriptase-2 cleavage of proteins		
TMPRSS6 autocleavage	PSSR↓IVGG	[8]
Hemojuvelin (furin site)	RNRRGAIT	[4; 13]
Fibronectin	single site	[8]
Type I collagen	single site	[8]
Fibrinogen	single site	[8]

Protein substrates and synthetic peptide substrates are listed. The cleavage sites are indicated with arrows (↓). The aa sequences of fibronectin, collagen, and fibrinogen do not reveal an obvious site that would be a target for matriptase-2.

CUB domains are found in mostly developmentally regulated proteins. Cubulin, which contains 27 CUB domains, has been shown to bind transferrin, hemoglobin, albumin, intrinsic factor-vitamin B_{12}, vitamin-D-binding protein, apolipoprotein A_1, and high-density lipoprotein, and participates in the processing of many of these proteins [5]. Binding of transferrin and hemoglobin to cubulin has been associated with transport into endosomes and lysosomes [5]. The CUB domain of platelet and endothelial cell surface protein SCUBE1 has been shown to bind BMP2 and plays a role in the secretion of mature BMP2 into the media [6]. The metalloproteinase ADAMTS13 contains two CUB domains, of which naturally occurring disease-associated mutations in the CUB1 domain have been identified. The mutations in the CUB1 domain of ADAMTS13 impaired secretion and stability of the secreted protease [7]. Of the two CUB domains in matriptase-2, the first one is degenerate relative to consensus CUB domains [8]. Nevertheless, it is likely that the CUB domains in matriptase-2 play a role in its own cell surface localization, and in substrate binding and processing. It has not been elucidated whether the CUB domains in matriptase-2 are able to bind transferrin or BMP2, two relevant proteins in iron homeostasis.

LDLa domains are cysteine-rich domains of approximately 40 aa with a conserved D/NXSDE motif of which the aspartic acid and glutamic acid residues are involved in calcium binding. LDLa domains have been found in a variety of functionally unrelated proteins and apparently play a role in the binding, internalization, and processing of proteins [9–11]. To date, matriptase-2 has not been shown to participate in the internalization of macromolecules, including substrates or substrate cleavage products, or mediate the processing of substrates within endocytic compartments, observed with some LDL receptor family members. Furthermore, it has not been determined if internalization or binding to matriptase-2 induces a signaling event.

Matriptase-2 Substrates

Autoactivation of matriptase-2 is predicted to occur by cleaving a conserved RIVGG motif located in the activation domain [8]. Matriptase-2 has been shown to cleave fibronectin, type 1 collagen, fibrinogen, pro-urokinase plasminogen activator, and artificial substrates with the peptide recognition sequence QAR and QGR [8] (table 1). Studies comparing substrate specificities of matriptase-2 to matriptase-1, hepsin and DESC1 demonstrated that matriptase-2 was the most promiscuous of the four proteases [12]. Matriptase-2 mediated efficient cleavage of artificial peptides corresponding to cleavage sites located in the proteins filaggrin, CUB-domain-containing protein 1 (CDCP1; also called transmembrane and associated with src kinases, Trask), and $α_E β_7$ integrin [12] (table 1). Using internally quenched fluorescent peptides as substrates, matriptase-2 demonstrated a preference for arginines in the P1 position and a basic aa in the P4 position. Matriptase-2 accommodates glycine, serine, alanine, isoleucine, or arginine in the P1′ position (table 1).

Hemojuvelin was the first biologically relevant exogenous substrate for matriptase-2 to be identified [4] (table 1). Coexpression of matriptase-2 with hemojuvelin resulted in the generation of several 25- to 30-kDa fragments and the reduction of all soluble hemojuvelin cleavage products at high concentrations of matriptase-2. Examination of the hemojuvelin sequence reveals the presence of a furin cleavage motif RNRR↓G that closely resembles the matriptase cleavage motif for filaggrin (RKR↓R↓GSRG). Nevertheless, the hemojuvelin R335Q mutant that alters the furin cleavage motif of hemojuvelin to RNRQG is cleaved in the same manner as wild-type hemojuvelin [4]. Although it is conceivable that matriptase-2 cleaves between arginine and glutamine of the R335Q mutant hemojuvelin (RNR↓Q) since the artificial peptide BocQNR-Amc is cleaved efficiently, the presence of a negatively charged aa (glutamic acid) at P4 and the glutamine at P1′ argue against this hypothesis [12]. Fur-

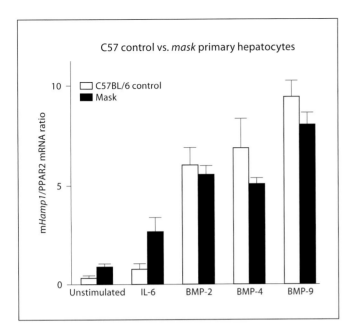

Fig. 2. Responsiveness of endogenous *Hamp1* mRNA expression to IL-6 and BMPs. Endogenous *Hamp1* expression was measured in primary hepatocytes isolated from matriptase-2 *mask* mutant or C57BL/6 control mice and stimulated with or without 10 ng/ml of IL-6, BMP2, BMP4, or BMP9. The normalization gene used is S18 ribosomal protein (PPAR2, GenBank accession No. AK050626). Each bar represents the mean ± SEM of two or three experiments each performed in triplicate.

thermore, the cleavage products of hemojuvelin mediated by matriptase-2 appear to differ from cleavage products of hemojuvelin mediated by furin [13]. Proteomic studies need to be performed to identify the sites of cleavage of hemojuvelin to determine if matriptase-2-mediated cleavage products are identical to previously described 'shed' hemojuvelin [14].

Matriptase-2 and Iron Homeostasis

The importance of matriptase-2 in iron homeostasis was first demonstrated by Du et al. [15] in mutant *mask* mice (MGI:3776631), generated by N-ethyl-N-nitrosourea mutagenesis [16]. *Mask* mice named for their truncal alopecia exhibited microcytic anemia, low plasma iron levels, low spleen iron stores, and high levels of *Hamp1* expression, inappropriate in the context of iron deficiency anemia [16]. The high expression of *Hamp1* mRNA, encoding the 25-aa iron-regulatory peptide hepcidin, accounted for the reduced intestinal iron absorption ob-

served in these mice [16]. *Mask* mice do not lower *Hamp1* mRNA levels in response to an iron-deficient diet as do C57 control mice [16]. Surprisingly, *mask* mice also do not increase *Hamp1* mRNA levels in response to a high-iron diet presumably because the higher than normal *Hamp1* mRNA levels reflect that mice are already 'seeing' an apparently high iron state [31]. Nevertheless, high dietary or parenteral iron levels are able to correct the low hemoglobin levels, alopecia, and female infertility in *Tmprss6 mask* mutant and null mice [16, 32]. Although *Hamp1* mRNA expression is unresponsive to iron in *mask* mice, *Hamp1* mRNA expression is responsive to stimulation by BMP2, BMP4, and BMP9, and to IL-6 (fig. 2).

Overexpression of wild-type or mutant (*mask* or the S762A) matriptase-2 in HepG2 cells demonstrated that wild-type but not mutant matriptase-2 repressed *Hamp1* reporter expression induced by BMP2, BMP9, IL-6, and hemojuvelin [16]. Thus, the in vitro data and the *mask* mouse phenotype supported that matriptase-2 was a potent inhibitor of *Hamp1* mRNA expression.

Overexpression of mutant (*mask* or R774C) matriptase-2 in zebrafish resulted in defective hemoglobin production suggesting a dominant negative effect over endogenous wild-type matriptase-2 [4]. Overexpression of wild-type matriptase-2 in zebrafish did not affect hemoglobin production, but it is not known whether the fish exhibited decreased *Hamp1* mRNA levels, increased ferroportin levels, and an iron overload phenotype compared to control fish [4].

The discovery of severe iron deficiency anemia in *mask* mice led to the identification of mutations in *TMPRSS6* in human patients with iron-refractory iron deficiency anemia (IRIDA) [17–20, 30]. In both mice and humans, the iron deficiency associated with mutations in *TMPRSS6* showed a recessive mode of transmission. Since the *Tmprss6–/–* mice (Tmprss6[tm1Otin], MGI:3809291) exhibited the identical iron deficiency phenotype, it is unlikely that mutations in *TMPRSS6* are associated with a gain-in-function phenotype. *Tmprss6–/–* mice exhibited reduced ferroportin immunostaining and iron accumulation in intestinal enterocytes consistent with a phenotype expected by overexpression of hepcidin [32].

The identification of hemojuvelin as a key substrate for matriptase-2 provided an explanation for the iron deficiency anemia associated with mutations in the gene for matriptase-2 *(TMPRSS6)* [4]. Cell surface hemojuvelin is correlated with hepcidin expression in hepatocytes [21]. Hemojuvelin is a coreceptor for some BMPs, in particular

BMP6, and participates in the activation of the SMAD1/ SMAD4 pathway to upregulate transcription of the hepcidin gene (HAMP) [22, 23, 33]. Deficiency in hemojuvelin, associated with juvenile hemochromatosis in humans, results in abnormally low expression of hepcidin leading to severe iron overload [24]. In matriptase-2 deficiency, hemojuvelin expression is presumably elevated leading to increased hepcidin expression, yet this remains to be demonstrated in vivo. Nevertheless, if this is the case, it is important to note that matriptase-2-deficient mice are not hyperresponsive to stimulation by BMP2, BMP4, or BMP9 (fig. 2).

Immunoprecipitation studies demonstrated physical association of matriptase-2 with hemojuvelin [4]. Binding to hemojuvelin occurred independently of the protease domain since the mask mutant matriptase-2 was also able to bind hemojuvelin. Coexpression of wild-type matriptase-2 and hemojuvelin in Hep3B or HeLa cells demonstrated cleavage of hemojuvelin. Matriptase-2 lacking or defective in the protease domain was unable to cleave hemojuvelin. Membrane-associated matriptase-2 does not cleave soluble hemojuvelin, and soluble matriptase does not cleave membrane-associated hemojuvelin. The data suggest that coexpression of matriptase-2 and membrane-associated hemojuvelin is required for cleavage [4].

In an effort to determine the phenotype of mice lacking both functional matriptase-2 and hemojuvelin, a double-mutant mouse strain $Hfe2^{tm1Nca/tm1Nca};Tmprss6^{Msk/Msk}$ was generated [31]. Mice lacking both matriptase-2 and hemojuvelin exhibited high plasma iron, high transferrin saturation, and normal hemoglobin and mean corpuscular volume, high liver iron content, and low $Hamp1$ mRNA levels, similar to hemojuvelin null mice. These data demonstrated that in the absence of both the positive and negative stimuli of hemojuvelin and matriptase-2, respectively, $Hamp1$ expression was constitutively off. Furthermore, $Hamp1$ mRNA expression in mice lacking both matriptase-2 and hemojuvelin was responsive to BMP2, BMP4, and BMP9, and the inflammatory cytokine IL-6, but was not responsive to high dietary iron. Therefore, mice lacking both matriptase-2 and hemojuvelin, being highly similar to hemojuvelin null mice, support the model that hemojuvelin is a substrate for matriptase-2. If matriptase-2 were acting on a substrate downstream of hemojuvelin, an iron-deficient or normal phenotype rather than an iron overload phenotype would have resulted.

Mutations and Polymorphisms in Matriptase-2

Mutations in matriptase-2 have provided insight into the mechanism of action of matriptase-2. Mutations associated with severe iron deficiency in mice or human patients predominately affect the proteolytic activity of matriptase-2 (fig. 1). Severe mutations in the protease domain of matriptase-2 causing premature termination and leading to an iron deficiency phenotype include the splice site mutation in mask mice (ivs14-2 A→G; C566fs) which deletes the entire protease domain, an R599X point mutation identified in zorro mice (Bruce Beutler, $Tmprss6^{m2Btlr}$, MGI:3812005) [25] and in an IRIDA patient [18], the W783X point mutation in masquerade mice (Bruce Beutler, $Tmprss6^{m3Btlr}$, MGI:3829007) [26], two deletion/insertion mutations A605fs, K636fs, and a splice site mutation (ivs16+1 G→C; G713fs) identified in IRIDA patients [17]. In addition, the point mutation identified in an IRIDA patient R774C located in the protease domain likely disrupts accurate C32/C36 or C35/C37 disulfide bonding within the protease domain [17]. Furthermore, the protease dead mutation, S762A in matriptase-2, has been shown in vitro to be ineffective in repressing $Hamp1$ reporter expression [16].

Point mutations D521N and E522K located in the conserved D/NXSDE motif in the LDLa2 domain of matriptase-2 have been associated with IRIDA in patients and affect residues predicted to bind Ca^{2+} [17, 20]. In vitro, the D521N and E522K mutants show reduced cell surface localization, increased Golgi retention, impaired autoactivation of matriptase-2, impaired cleavage of hemojuvelin, and impaired ability to repress $Hamp1$ reporter expression but are able to bind hemojuvelin [20].

Matriptase-2 containing the point mutation G442R located in the second CUB domain demonstrated impaired autoactivation, was still able to bind but demonstrated reduced cleavage of coexpressed hemojuvelin, and exhibited reduced ability to repress $HAMP$ reporter expression [20].

The mutants L166fs and S288fs result in severe truncation of the ectodomain and if they localize to the cell surface, they are likely to be severely impaired in their ability to bind hemojuvelin. These mutations identified in homozygous IRIDA patients suggest that loss of proteolytic cleavage of hemojuvelin rather than increased stabilization or retention of hemojuvelin on the cell surface by mutant matriptase-2 is sufficient to cause the IRIDA phenotype. Furthermore, these data demonstrate that homozygous loss of the bulk of the ectodomain does not induce

Table 2. List of coding region polymorphisms in the human TMPRSS6 gene

SNP ID	Genomic coordinates	Contiguous coordinates	Alleles	Coding coordinates	AA	NCBI allele frequency
	129	16890080	C/T	15	F5F	
rs11704654	308	16889901	A/G	99	P33P	0.299
rs5756514	5198	16885011	C/T	323	**S108F**	ND
	13896	16876313	A/G	683	**G228D***	
rs35961386	13903	16876306	C/T	690	G230G	ND
rs2235324	13970	16876239	A/G	757	**K253E**	0.496
rs5995378	14076	16876133	C/T	863	S288L	0.034
rs2543517	17358	16872851	G/A	987	P329P	ND
rs2111833	18897	16871312	G/A	1083	S361S	0.452
rs881144	28404	16861805	C/T	1254	Y418Y	ND
	28486	16861723	C/T	1336	**R446W***	
rs4820268	30103	16860106	C/T	1563	D521D	0.488
rs855791	36758	16853451	T/C	2207	**V736A**	0.416
rs2235321	36768	16853441	C/T	2217	Y739Y	0.471
rs11703011	36826	16852783	G/A	2288	**G763D**	ND
rs73886915	36884	16852725	C/T	2346	S782S	ND
	37521	16852688	A/G	2383	**V795I***	ND

Coding region polymorphisms identified in the NCBI SNP database, or by screening (*) of subjects with or without iron deficiency anemia of unknown etiology [30]. ND = Not determined.

an intracellular signal leading to repression of hepcidin expression, as previously proposed [16].

Thus most, if not all of the disease-associated mutations in *TMPRSS6*, result in the loss of proteolytic activity by loss of the protease domain or reduction in autoactivation, or in a reduction in cell surface localization.

The identification of severe mutations in matriptase-2 associated with IRIDA raised the question as to whether mild mutations or polymorphisms might contribute to iron deficiency anemia in patients lacking predisposing factors. Examination of the TMPRSS6 gene revealed that the gene was highly polymorphic, particularly in noncoding regions. Coding region polymorphisms occurring in the general population (table 2) did not appear to correlate with iron deficiency anemia of no known etiology, although the allele frequencies of rare polymorphisms located in highly conserved regions of the protein were too low to establish statistical significance [30]. Nevertheless, in one family study, the presence of an uncommon R446W polymorphism in trans with a severe TMPRSS6 mutation appeared to be associated with ironresponsive iron deficiency anemia. Functional studies need to be performed to determine if these rare polymorphisms in matriptase-2 exhibit impaired hemojuvelin degradation and impaired suppression of *Hamp1* expression.

Hemojuvelin Shedding

How does liver-specific matriptase-2 fit into the earlier reports of soluble hemojuvelin in cell culture supernatants, serum, and plasma [21]? Previously, the release of hemojuvelin into cell culture media was shown to be suppressed by transferrin-bound iron or ferric ammonium citrate [21]. Soluble hemojuvelin is biologically active as a competitive inhibitor that can antagonize the binding of BMPs to the BMP receptor [21]. Is the cleavage of hemojuvelin by matriptase-2 sensitive to iron? Are the products of hemojuvelin by matriptase-2 cleavage able to antagonize BMP binding? When HeLa cells are cotransfected with matriptase-2 and hemojuvelin, multiple cleavage products of hemojuvelin and loss of soluble hemojuvelin are observed [4], suggesting that the function of matriptase-2 is to degrade hemojuvelin rather than to produce an antagonist, but this remains to be examined in greater experimental detail.

Kuninger et al. [27], Zhang et al. [28], and Lin et al. [21] demonstrated independently that hemojuvelin is shed from muscle cells (C2C12), transfected liver (HepG2 and Hep3B), and kidney cells (HEK293), strongly suggesting that there are matriptase-2-dependent and -independent pathways for shedding hemojuvelin since matriptase-2 is almost exclusively expressed in the liver. Kuninger et al. [27] demonstrated that cell surface biotin-labeled hemojuvelin could be shed from the cell surface. The shed hemojuvelin was primarily of the form uncleaved at the 172Asp-173Pro bond. Lin et al. [14] demonstrated that hemojuvelin released from transfected HEK293 cells was cleaved by a furin-like proprotein convertase at the furin site and included both 172Asp-173Pro-cleaved and uncleaved forms of hemojuvelin. In the presence of inhibitors of furin-like proteases, hemojuvelin was shed from the cell surface by an alternative pathway, possibly by the action of phopholipase A, cleaving the glycosylphosphatidylinositol anchor and releasing the entire hemojuvelin ectodomain [14].

Silvestri et al. [13] demonstrated that mutants of hemojuvelin that were retained in the endoplasmic reticulum still released soluble hemojuvelin despite reduced cell surface localization, suggesting that soluble hemojuvelin was secreted from the endoplasmic reticulum rather than shed from the cell surface. Furthermore, they also provided evidence that cleavage of hemojuvelin was mediated by the protease furin which was transcriptionally regulated by iron and hypoxia. Cotransfection of HeLa and HepG2 cells with furin and hemojuvelin did not appear to show the same cleavage products as cotransfection with matriptase-2 and hemojuvelin [13].

Zhang et al. [28] indicated that hemojuvelin shedding is regulated by neogenin. Coexpression of hemojuvelin with neogenin in HepG2 cells increased hemojuvelin shedding. Likewise, knockdown of endogenous neogenin in C2C12 cells transfected with hemojuvelin suppressed hemojuvelin shedding. Coexpression of hemojuvelin with neogenin in HEK293 cells was associated with increased iron loading [29].

The data seem to indicate that there are several pathways by which hemojuvelin can be released from cells, more than one of which may be sensitive to iron regulation. If this is the case, they clearly are not redundant since they do not compensate for the loss of matriptase-2 in humans and mice. Matriptase-2-independent shedding of hemojuvelin does not result in a major change in cell surface levels of hemojuvelin [13, 28] and appears to function to generate a soluble antagonist that can act in an autocrine or paracrine fashion depending on the tissue source, be it hepatocytes or muscles. In contrast, matriptase-2-dependent cleavage results in a major loss of hemojuvelin from the hepatocyte cell surface [4], and its function appears to be removal of the positive effect cell-associated hemojuvelin has on hepcidin expression. Removal of cell-associated hemojuvelin has a dominant phenotype over the antagonistic function of soluble hemojuvelin.

Transcriptional Regulation of Matriptase-2

The transcriptional regulation of matriptase-2 might provide insight into mediators of matriptase-2 expression that indirectly effect iron homeostasis. Comparison of the genomic organization and nucleotide sequences of exons 1, 5′-untranslated regions and proximal promoter regions of the human and murine TMPRSS6 genes demonstrated that these regions are not conserved between species (fig. 3). Examination of the predicted transcription factor binding sites by Genomatix MatInspector (http://www.genomatix.com) identified a krueppel-like C2H2 zinc finger factor hypermethylated in cancer (HIC1) motif, a peroxisome proliferator-activated receptor (PPAR_RXR) motif, a nuclear receptor subfamily 2 factor (COUP) motif, a pancreas transcription factor 1, a heterotrimeric transcription factor (PTFI) motif, and an NKX homeodomain factor (NKXH) motif in common between human and murine proximal promoters, but currently there is no known biological relevance for any of these transcription factors in the regulation of matriptase-2 expression (fig. 3).

Since hepcidin expression is repressed by hypoxia and anemia, it raises the question whether matriptase-2 plays a role in this repression. Studies need to be performed to examine if transcriptional and posttranscriptional regulation of matriptase-2 by hypoxia or iron deficiency might contribute indirectly to the repression of hepcidin.

Summary and Future Perspectives

The current working model for the role of matriptase-2 in iron homeostasis has membrane-anchored matriptase-2 as an active protease acting as the central modulator of hemojuvelin cell surface expression (fig. 4a). Cleavage of hemojuvelin results in loss from the hepatocyte cell surface and the loss of hemojuvelin to act as a coreceptor for BMPs. Nevertheless, BMPs can still upregulate hepci-

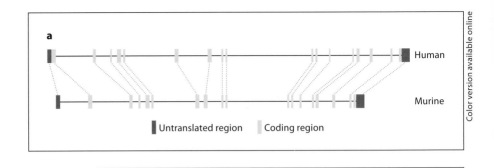

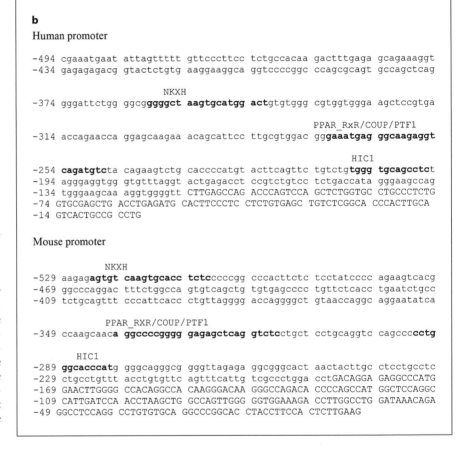

Fig. 3. Analysis of the human and murine *TMPRSS6* genes. **a** Alignment of the genomic organization of the human and murine *TMPRSS6* genes. **b** Genomatix MatInspector predicted transcription factor motifs common in the proximal promoter regions of the human and murine TMPRSS6 genes. The genomic organization at the 5′ ends of the human and murine genes is not conserved. There is little to no sequence homology between the human and murine promoter and 5′-untranslated regions. Non-coding genomic coordinates are used (numbering from the ATG).

din expression directly through the BMP receptors in the absence of hemojuvelin. Likewise, inflammatory cytokines such as IL-6 are able to upregulate hepcidin expression in the absence of hemojuvelin. It remains to be determined if matriptase-2-mediated cleavage products of hemojuvelin are able to act as a soluble antagonist for the binding of BMPs to the cognate receptor in the same manner as soluble hemojuvelin [21]. The matriptase-2 *mask* mutant lacking the protease domain is able to localize to the cell surface and can bind hemojuvelin. Uncleaved hemojuvelin is stable and retained on the cell sur-

face where it is perpetually available to promote BMP-mediated activation of hepcidin expression. The presence of the matriptase-2 *mask* mutant does not interfere with IL-6-mediated upregulation of hepcidin expression (fig. 4b).

There are so many questions left to answer, many of which were raised throughout the manuscript. Is matriptase-2 activity regulated by iron? What roles do TfR2, HFE, and neogenin play, if any, to relay the iron status to matriptase-2? If matriptase-2 is not regulated by iron then what is it regulated by – hypoxia? Are there multiple

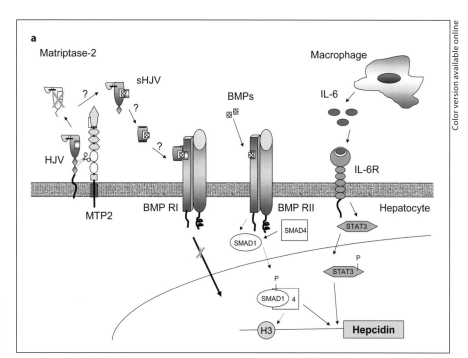

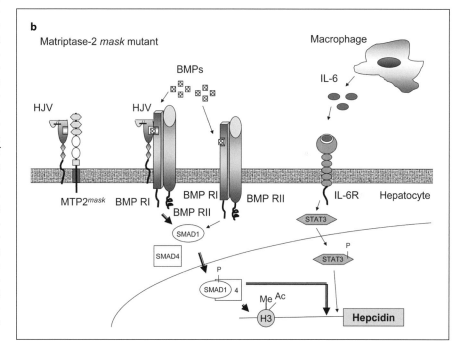

Fig. 4. Working model of matriptase-2 regulation of iron homeostasis. **a** Membrane-anchored matriptase-2 (MTP2) is an active protease cleaving hemojuvelin (HJV) resulting in loss of hemojuvelin, a coreceptor for BMPs, from the hepatocyte cell surface. Nevertheless, BMPs can still upregulate hepcidin expression directly through binding to the BMP receptors in the absence of hemojuvelin. Likewise, inflammatory cytokines such as IL-6 are able to upregulate hepcidin expression in the absence of hemojuvelin. It remains to be determined if matriptase-2-mediated cleavage products of hemojuvelin are able to act as a soluble antagonist for the binding of BMPs to the cognate receptor in the same manner as soluble hemojuvelin (sHJV). **b** The matriptase-2 *mask* (MTP2^{mask}) mutant lacking the protease domain is able to localize to the cell surface and can bind hemojuvelin. Uncleaved hemojuvelin is stable and retained on the cell surface where it is perpetually available to promote BMP-mediated activation of hepcidin expression. The presence of the matriptase-2 *mask* mutant does not interfere with IL-6-mediated upregulation of hepcidin expression.

pathways for cleaving hemojuvelin – a shedding pathway to produce a soluble antagonist and another to degrade cell surface hemojuvelin?

Are there other biologically important substrates for matriptase-2? Does soluble matriptase-2 (shed from the cell surface) have physiological importance?

Acknowledgments

This work (manuscript 20141-MEM from the Scripps Research Institute) was supported by grants from the National Institutes of Health (grant DK53505-10), the Skaggs Scholars in Clinical Science Program from the Scripps Research Institute and the Stein Endowment Fund.

References

1 Ramsay AJ, Hooper JD, Folgueras AR, Velasco G, Lopez-Otin C: Matriptase-2 (TMPRSS6): a proteolytic regulator of iron homeostasis. Haematologica 2009;94:840–849.

2 Knutson MD: Into the matrix: regulation of the iron regulatory hormone hepcidin by matriptase-2. Nutr Rev 2009;67:284–288.

3 Muckenthaler MU: Fine tuning of hepcidin expression by positive and negative regulators. Cell Metab 2008;8:1–3.

4 Silvestri L, Pagani A, Nai A, De Domenico I, Kaplan J, Camaschella C: The serine protease matriptase-2 (TMPRSS6) inhibits hepcidin activation by cleaving membrane hemojuvelin. Cell Metab 2008;8:502–511.

5 Christensen EI, Birn H: Megalin and cubilin: multifunctional endocytic receptors. Nat Rev Mol Cell Biol 2002;3:256–266.

6 Tu CF, Yan YT, Wu SY, Djoko B, Tsai MT, Cheng CJ, Yang RB: Domain and functional analysis of a novel platelet-endothelial cell surface protein, SCUBE1. J Biol Chem 2008;283:12478–12488.

7 Zhou Z, Jing H, Tao Z, Choi H, Aboulfatova K, Moake J, Li R, Dong JF: Effects of naturally occurring mutations in CUB-1 domain on synthesis, stability, and activity of AD-AMTS-13. Thromb Res 2009;124:323–327.

8 Velasco G, Cal S, Quesada A, Sanchez LM, Lopez-Otin C: Matriptase-2, a membrane-bound mosaic serine proteinase predominantly expressed in human liver and showing degrading activity against extracellular matrix proteins. J Biol Chem 2002;277:37637–37646.

9 Horn IR, van den Berg BM, Moestrup SK, Pannekoek H, van Zonneveld AJ: Plasminogen activator inhibitor 1 contains a cryptic high affinity receptor binding site that is exposed upon complex formation with tissue-type plasminogen activator. Thromb Haemost 1998;80:822–828.

10 Cam JA, Bu G: Modulation of beta-amyloid precursor protein trafficking and processing by the low density lipoprotein receptor family. Mol Neurodegener 2006;1:8.

11 Parkyn CJ, Vermeulen EG, Mootoosamy RC, Sunyach C, Jacobsen C, Oxvig C, Moestrup S, Liu Q, Bu G, Jen A, Morris RJ: LRP1 controls biosynthetic and endocytic trafficking of neuronal prion protein. J Cell Sci 2008;121:773–783.

12 Beliveau F, Desilets A, Leduc R: Probing the substrate specificities of matriptase, matriptase-2, hepsin and DESC1 with internally quenched fluorescent peptides. FEBS J 2009;276:2213–2226.

13 Silvestri L, Pagani A, Camaschella C: Furin-mediated release of soluble hemojuvelin: a new link between hypoxia and iron homeostasis. Blood 2008;111:924–931.

14 Lin L, Nemeth E, Goodnough JB, Thapa DR, Gabayan V, Ganz T: Soluble hemojuvelin is released by proprotein convertase-mediated cleavage at a conserved polybasic RNRR site. Blood Cells Mol Dis 2008;40:122–131.

15 Du X, Moresco EMY, Beutler B: Tmprss6 mask (updated 9-28-2008). La Jolla, Mutagenetix, accessed 5-10-09. http://mutagenetix.scripps.edu.

16 Du X, She E, Gelbart T, Truksa J, Lee P, Xia Y, Khovananth K, Mudd S, Mann N, Moresco EM, Beutler E, Beutler B: The serine protease TMPRSS6 is required to sense iron deficiency. Science 2008;320:1088–1092.

17 Finberg KE, Heeney MM, Campagna DR, Aydinok Y, Pearson HA, Hartman KR, Mayo MM, Samuel SM, Strouse JJ, Markianos K, Andrews NC, Fleming MD: Mutations in TMPRSS6 cause iron-refractory iron deficiency anemia (IRIDA). Nat Genet 2008;40:569–571.

18 Guillem F, Lawson S, Kannengiesser C, Westerman M, Beaumont C, Grandchamp B: Two nonsense mutations in the TMPRSS6 gene in a patient with microcytic anemia and iron deficiency. Blood 2008;112:2089–2091.

19 Melis MA, Cau M, Congiu R, Sole G, Barella S, Cao A, Westerman M, Cazzola M, Galanello R: A mutation in the TMPRSS6 gene, encoding a transmembrane serine protease that suppresses hepcidin production, in familial iron deficiency anemia refractory to oral iron. Haematologica 2008;93:1473–1479.

20 Silvestri L, Guillem F, Pagani A, Nai A, Oudin C, Silva M, Toutain F, Kannengiesser C, Beaumont C, Camaschella C, Grandchamp B: Molecular mechanisms of the defective hepcidin inhibition in TMPRSS6 mutations associated with iron-refractory iron deficiency anemia. Blood 2009;113:5605–5608.

21 Lin L, Goldberg YP, Ganz T: Competitive regulation of hepcidin mRNA by soluble and cell-associated hemojuvelin. Blood 2005;106:2884–2889.

22 Huang FW, Babitt JL, Wrighting DM, Samad TA, Xia Y, Sidis Y, Campagna JA, Chung RT, Schneyer AL, Woolf CJ, Andrews NC, Lin HY: Hemojuvelin acts as a bone morphogenetic protein co-receptor to regulate hepcidin. Blood 2005;106:153a.

23 Meynard D, Kautz L, Darnaud V, Canonne-Hergaux F, Coppin H, Roth MP: Lack of the bone morphogenetic protein BMP6 induces massive iron overload. Nat Genet 2009;41:478–481.

24 Papanikolaou G, Samuels ME, Ludwig EH, MacDonald ML, Franchini PL, Dube MP, Andres L, MacFarlane J, Sakellaropoulos N, Politou M, Nemeth E, Thompson J, Risler JK, Zaborowska C, Babakaiff R, Radomski CC, Pape TD, Davidas O, Christakis J, Brissot P, Lockitch G, Ganz T, Hayden MR, Goldberg YP: Mutations in HFE2 cause iron overload in chromosome 1q-linked juvenile hemochromatosis. Nat Genet 2004;36:77–82.

25 Du X, Moresco EMY, Beutler B: Tmprss6 zorro (updated 9-28-2008). La Jolla, Mutagenetix, accessed 5-10-09. http://mutagenetix.scripps.edu.

26 Du X, Moresco EMY, Beutler B: Tmprss6 masquerade (9-28-2008). La Jolla, Mutagenix, accessed 5-10-09. http://mutagenetix.scripps.edu.

27 Kuninger D, Kuns-Hashimoto R, Kuzmickas R, Rotwein P: Complex biosynthesis of the muscle-enriched iron regulator RGMc. J Cell Sci 2006;119:3273–3283.

28 Zhang AS, Anderson SA, Meyers KR, Hernandez C, Eisenstein RS, Enns CA: Evidence that inhibition of hemojuvelin shedding in response to iron is mediated through neogenin. J Biol Chem 2007;282:12547–12556.

29 Zhang AS, West AP Jr, Wyman AE, Bjorkman PJ, Enns CA: Interaction of hemojuvelin with neogenin results in iron accumulation in human embryonic kidney 293 cells. J Biol Chem 2005;280:33885–33894.

30 Beutler E, Van Geet C, Te Loo DM, Gelbart T, Crain K, Truksa J, Lee PL: Polymorphisms and mutations of human TMPRSS6 in iron deficiency anemia. Blood Cells Mol Dis 2009; in press.

31 Truksa J, Gelbart T, Peng H, Beutler E, Beutler B, Lee P: Suppression of the hepcidin-encoding gene Hamp permits iron overload in mice lacking both hemojuvelin and matriptase-2/TMPRSS6. Brit J Haematol DOI:10.1111/j.1365-2141.2009.07873x.

32 Folgueras AR, de Lara FM, Pendas AM, Garabaya C, Rodriguez F, Astudillo A, Bernal T, Cabanillas R, Lopez-Otin C, Velasco G: Membrane-bound serine protease matriptase-2 (Tmprss6) is an essential regulator of iron homeostasis. Blood 2008;112:2539–2545.

33 Andriopoulos B Jr, Corradini E, Xia Y, Faasse SA, Chen S, Grgurevic L, Knutson MD, Pietrangelo A, Vukicevic S, Lin HY, Babitt JL: BMP6 is a key endogenous regulator of hepcidin expression and iron metabolism. Nat Genet DOI:10.1038/ng.335.

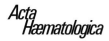

Acta Haematol 2009;122:97–102
DOI: 10.1159/000243793

Published online: November 10, 2009

Iron Deficiency, *Helicobacter* Infection and Gastritis

Chaim Hershko[a, b]   Aharon Ronson[a, c]

[a]Department of Hematology, Shaare Zedek Medical Center, [b]Hematology Clinic and Central Clinical Laboratories, Clalit Health Services, and [c]Hematology Clinics, Meuhedet Health Services, Jerusalem, Israel

Key Words
Autoimmune atrophic gastritis · Celiac disease · Gastritis · *Helicobacter* · Iron deficiency anemia · Vitamin B_{12}

Abstract
Despite elegant regulatory mechanisms, iron deficiency anemia (IDA) remains one of the most common nutritional deficiencies of mankind. Iron deficiency is the result of an interplay between increased host requirements, limited external supply, and increased blood loss. When related to increased physiologic needs associated with normal development, iron deficiency is designated physiologic or nutritional. By contrast, pathological iron deficiency, with the exception of gross menorrhagia, is most often the result of gastrointestinal disease associated with abnormal blood loss or malabsorption. If gastroenterologic evaluation fails to disclose a likely cause of IDA, or in patients refractory to oral iron treatment, screening for celiac disease (anti-tissue transglutaminase antibodies), autoimmune gastritis (gastrin, antiparietal or anti-intrinsic factor antibodies), and *Helicobacter pylori* (IgG antibodies and urease breath test) is recommended. Recent studies indicate that 20–27% of patients with unexplained IDA have autoimmune gastritis, about 50% have evidence of active *H. pylori* infection, and 4–6% have celiac disease. The implications for abnormal iron absorption of celiac disease or autoimmune gastritis are obvious. In patients with unexplained IDA and *H. pylori* infection, cure of refractory IDA by *H. pylori* eradication offers strong evidence for a cause-and-effect relation between *H. pylori* infection and unexplained IDA. Stratification by age cohorts in autoimmune gastritis implies a disease presenting as IDA many years before the establishment of clinical cobalamin deficiency. It is likely caused by an autoimmune process triggered by antigenic mimicry between *H. pylori* epitopes and major autoantigens of the gastric mucosa. Recognition of the respective roles of *H. pylori* and autoimmune gastritis in the pathogenesis of iron deficiency may have a strong impact on the diagnostic workup and management of unexplained, or refractory IDA.

Copyright © 2009 S. Karger AG, Basel

Introduction

As a transition metal, iron plays an essential role in life by its ability to accept and donate electrons. Some of the most important functions of iron proteins are oxygen transport, mitochondrial oxidative energy production, inactivation of drugs and toxins, and DNA synthesis. The solubility of iron in its stable, oxidized form is extremely low and, although iron is one of the most abundant elements in nature, paradoxically iron deficiency is one of the most common nutritional problems of the human race [1].

C. Hershko
Department Hematology
Shaare Zedek Medical Center, POB 3235
IL–91031 Jerusalem (Israel)
Tel. +972 2 655 5567, Fax +972 2 570 0693, E-Mail hershko@szmc.org.il

Mechanisms of Iron Deficiency

Despite the carefully orchestrated mechanism of normal iron homeostasis, iron deficiency is still a major health problem. Its development is the result of an interplay between three distinct risk factors: increased host requirements, limited external supply, and increased blood loss. Iron deficiency is associated with serious health risks, including abnormal mental and motor development in infancy; impaired work capacity; increased risk of premature delivery, and increased maternal and infant mortality in severe anemia [1].

Increased requirements are the result of increased physiologic needs associated with normal development. This category of iron deficiency is often designated *physiologic*, or nutritional. By contrast, *pathologic* iron deficiency, with the exception of gross menorrhagia, is most often the result of gastrointestinal (GI) disease associated with abnormal blood loss or malabsorption. Consequently, in grown males and postmenopausal females, complete gastroenterologic investigation is recommended to identify pathological lesions responsible for abnormal blood loss. However, conventional endoscopic and radiographic methods fail to identify a probable source of GI blood loss in about one third of males and postmenopausal females and in most young women with iron deficiency anemia (IDA) [2–4].

Obscure or Refractory Iron Deficiency

In recent years, there has been an increasing awareness of subtle, non-bleeding GI conditions that may result in abnormal iron absorption leading to IDA in the absence of GI symptoms. Thus, the importance of celiac disease as a possible cause of IDA refractory to oral iron treatment, without other apparent manifestations of malabsorption syndrome [5], is increasingly recognized. In addition, *Helicobacter pylori* has been implicated in several recent studies as a cause of IDA refractory to oral iron treatment, with a favorable response to *H. pylori* eradication [6, 7]. Likewise, autoimmune atrophic gastritis, a condition associated with chronic idiopathic iron deficiency, has been shown to be responsible for refractory IDA in over 20% of patients with no evidence of GI blood loss [8, 9]. Hereditary iron deficiency due to mutations in the serine protease matriptase-2 (TMPRSS6) has been discussed by Lee (pp 87–96) in another chapter of this issue.

The recent availability of convenient, non-invasive screening methods for identifying celiac disease (anti-tis-sue transglutaminase or TTG antibodies), autoimmune atrophic gastritis (serum gastrin/parietal cell antibodies) and *H. pylori* infection (antibody screening and urease breath test) greatly facilitated the recognition of patients with these entities, resulting in an increased awareness of these conditions and their possible role in the causation of IDA.

In a prospective study, we have screened 300 consecutive patients referred with unexplained or refractory IDA to a hematology outpatient clinic, employing the above methods for identifying non-bleeding GI conditions (table 1). The mean age of all subjects was 39 ± 18 years, and 251 of the 300 (84%) were women of reproductive age. We identified 18 new cases of *adult celiac disease* (6%). Seventy-seven IDA patients (26%) had *autoimmune atrophic gastritis* of whom 39 (51%) had coexistent *H. pylori* infection. *H. pylori* infection was the only finding in 57 patients (19%), but was a common coexisting finding in 165 (55%) of the entire group. Refractoriness to oral iron treatment was found in 100% of patients with celiac disease, 69% with autoimmune atrophic gastritis, 68% with *H. pylori* infection, but only 10% of subjects with no apparent underlying abnormality. In the following, we wish to discuss the implications of the above findings for the pathogenesis and management of 'unexplained' IDA.

Celiac Disease

IDA without other clinical clues of intestinal malabsorption is one of the most common extraintestinal manifestations of celiac disease [10, 11] reported in about 50% of patients with subclinical celiac disease. Conversely, among patients presenting with unexplained IDA, celiac disease is the underlying pathology responsible for anemia in 5–6% of cases [12–16]. Demonstration of histological changes in the small bowel mucosa is still regarded as the gold standard of diagnosis in celiac disease. However, the discovery of anti-endomysial antibodies in patients with celiac disease had a major impact on the subsequent evolution of screening and algorithms for diagnosing celiac disease [17]. Its specificity and sensitivity are estimated at 99 and >90%, respectively. More recently, an enzyme-linked immunosorbent assay has been developed to determine anti-TTG IgA antibody activity, and it is cheaper and more convenient, with sensitivity and specificity being comparable to the older anti-endomysial indirect fluorescence test. A characteristic feature of IDA associated with celiac disease is its refractoriness to oral iron treatment.

Table 1. Main diagnostic categories and coexistent findings in 300 IDA patients referred for hematologic evaluation

Diagnosis	Autoimmune atrophic gastritis	*H. pylori*	Menorrhagia	GI lesions	Celiac	Negative
Patients, n	77 (26%)	57 (19%)	96 (32%)	31 (10%)	18 (6%)	21 (7%)
Age, years	41 ± 16	37 ± 19	39 ± 10	60 ± 14	39 ± 14	33 ± 13
Gender, males/females	14/63	17/40	0/96	13/18	3/15	2/19
Main diagnosis alone	26	57	39	21	15	21
H. pylori	39	–	57	10	2	0
Menorrhagia	11	0	–	0	1	0
GI lesions	1	0	0	–	0	0
Aspirin or NSAID	9	3	1	7	0	1
Refractory to oral iron, %	69	68	38	47	100	10

In total, *H. pylori* infection was a coexistent finding in 165 patients. Use of aspirin or non-steroidal anti-inflammatory drugs (NSAID) is listed as additional information but is not counted separately in the total number of subjects. Under the heading 'celiac', 4 patients with gastroplasty are also included [50].

Autoimmune Atrophic Gastritis

The concept of gastric atrophy as a cause of IDA is not new. *Achylia gastrica* associated with IDA was first described as a clinical entity by Faber [18] in 1909, and *achlorhydric gastric atrophy*, a synonym for the same entity, has long been recognized as a major cause of IDA [19] but largely forgotten, and completely ignored in subsequent major surveys of GI causes of IDA. More recently, achlorhydric gastric atrophy has been rediscovered by Dickey et al. [9] and implicated in 20% of IDA patients with no evidence of GI blood loss. This observation was confirmed and greatly extended in a series of important studies by Annibale et al. [8], who found 27% of patients with refractory IDA without GI symptoms to have atrophic body gastritis, a percentage identical with the proportion of subjects with autoimmune atrophic body gastritis in our own studies [20]. Iron absorption is severely impaired in achylia gastrica, and impaired iron absorption in pernicious anemia is corrected by normal, but not by neutralized gastric juice, indicating that lack of gastric acidity is the key factor in abnormal iron absorption [21]. Other studies have also shown that iron absorption is heavily dependent on normal gastric secretion and acidity for solubilizing and reducing dietary iron [22, 23]. Although atrophic gastritis may impair both B_{12} and iron absorption simultaneously, in young women in whom menstruation represents an added strain on iron requirements, iron deficiency will develop many years before the depletion of vitamin B_{12} stores. With the subsequent loss of the remaining gastric parietal cells mediated by humoral and/or cellular autoimmunity, residual cobalamin stores will be completely depleted resulting in the full clinical manifestations of pernicious anemia.

H. pylori Gastritis

The role of *H. pylori* in the causation of IDA is of considerable current interest. Major population surveys involving thousands of subjects [24] conducted over diverse geographic areas all indicate that *H. pylori* positivity is associated with an increased prevalence of iron deficiency. Several population studies conducted in various regions of Alaska indicate that active *H. pylori* infection is independently associated with iron deficiency and IDA [25], and that a significant association between low serum ferritin levels and prevalence of *H.-pylori*-specific IgG exists, particularly among people aged <20 years. [26].The largest study of this category was performed among 7,462 survey participants aged >3 years from the 1999–2000 National Health and Nutrition Examination Survey. This study showed that in the United States, *H. pylori* infection diagnosed by serology is associated with a 40% increase in the prevalence of iron deficiency [27].

The most convincing evidence of a cause-and-effect relation between IDA and *H. pylori* infection is demonstration of the beneficial effects of *H. pylori* eradication on preexisting IDA. Such a beneficial effect has previously been shown in patients with duodenal ulcer, atrophy of the gastric body predisposing to gastric ulcer and cancer, and mucosa-associated lymphoid tissue lymphoma [28].

Well-documented clinical cases, mainly of children and adolescents, published as early as 1993, have shown that IDA (in particular iron-resistant anemia) could be corrected by eradication of *H. pylori*, even without associated iron supplementation [29].

Our own observations indicating that failure to respond to oral iron treatment in *H.-pylori*-positive patients was more than twice as common as in the *H.-pylori*-negative group, and that successful *H. pylori* eradication resulted in an increase in hemoglobin levels indistinguishable from that in previously responsive IDA patients [20], are in agreement with a number of previous studies [7, 30, 31]. Most of these reports involved young females refractory to oral iron treatment, and improvement has been observed following *H. pylori* eradication even in the absence of continued iron administration.

However, menstrual blood loss is a serious compounding factor in evaluating alternative causes of IDA. Consequently, in a subsequent study we have focused on 29 male IDA patients with negative GI workup and refractory to oral iron treatment. Twenty-five of the 29 patients had active *H. pylori* infection with or without coexistent *autoimmune gastritis* [32]. Following *H. pylori* eradication, all patients achieved normal hemoglobin levels with follow-up periods ranging from 4 to 69 months (38 ± 15 months, mean ± SD). This was accompanied by a significant decrease in *H. pylori* IgG antibodies and in serum gastrin levels. Sixteen patients discontinued iron treatment, maintaining normal hemoglobin and ferritin and may be considered cured. Remarkably, 4 of the 16 patients achieved normal hemoglobin without ever having received oral iron after *H. pylori* eradication.

A number of possible mechanisms have been invoked to explain the relation between *H. pylori* gastritis and IDA, including occult GI bleeding and competition for dietary iron by the bacteria. The late Ernie Beutler suggested that it might be possible for *H. pylori* to subvert the human iron regulatory mechanism in a manner that is beneficial to the microorganism but deleterious to the host. This could be achieved by the production of hepcidin mimics that prevent the response to iron [33]. An alternative hypothesis that would probably have been equally appealing to Ernie Beutler is the possibility that *H. pylori* produces inhibitors to matriptase interfering with the normal response of intestinal mucosa to iron depletion [34].

Occult GI bleeding is a likely cause in some patients, as suggested by the rapid relapse of their anemia that cannot be explained by impaired absorption alone. However, the most likely explanation is the effect of *H. pylori* on the composition of gastric juice. Studies in *H.-pylori*-positive subjects have shown decreased oral iron absorption reverting to normal after *H. pylori* eradication [35].

Absorption of iron necessitates a reduction in the ferric to ferrous form, which is dependent upon the pH of gastric juice and ascorbic acid. Studies by Annibale et al. [36] have shown that gastric acidity and ascorbate content, both of which are critical for normal iron absorption, are adversely affected by *H. pylori* infection and that *H. pylori* eradication results in normalization of intragastric pH and ascorbate content.

Possible role of *H. pylori* in the Pathogenesis of Autoimmune Gastritis

With an intent to define the relation between IDA associated with autoimmune gastritis and pernicious anemia, we have studied 160 patients with autoimmune gastritis of whom 83 presented with IDA, 48 with autoimmune gastritis and normocytic indices, and 29 with macrocytic anemia [37]. Stratification by age cohorts of autoimmune gastritis from <20 to >60 years showed a prevalence of coexistent *H. pylori* infection in 87.5% aged <20 years, 47% 20–40 years, 37.5% 41–60 years and 12.5% aged >60 years. With age increasing from <20 to >60 years, there was a regular and progressive increase in mean corpuscular volume from 68 ± 9 to 95 ± 16 fl, serum ferritin from 4 ± 2 to 37 ± 41 μg/l, and gastrin from 349 ± 247 to 800 ± 627 U/ml, and a decrease in cobalamin from 392 ± 179 to 108 ± 65 pg/ml.

Survival of *H. pylori* requires an acid environment that no longer exists in advanced gastric atrophy. The high prevalence of *H. pylori* positivity in young patients with autoimmune gastritis and its almost total absence in elderly patients with pernicious anemia implies that *H. pylori* infection in autoimmune gastritis may represent an early phase of disease in which an infectious process is gradually replaced by an autoimmune disease terminating in burned-out infection and the irreversible destruction of gastric body mucosa. Although this question has long intrigued investigators, the relation between *H. pylori* and the pathogenesis of pernicious anemia is still unsettled [38]. *H.-pylori*-infected subjects have circulating IgG antibodies directed against epitopes on gastric mucosal cells. Of these, the most likely target of an autoimmune mechanism triggered by *H. pylori* and directed against gastric parietal cells by means of antigenic mimicry [39–42] is H^+K^+-ATPase, a protein that is the most common autoantigen in pernicious anemia. Conversely,

H. pylori eradication in patients with autoimmune atrophic gastritis is followed by improved gastric acid and ascorbate secretion in many, and complete remission of atrophic gastritis in a variable proportion of patients [43–45]. However, the rate of histological improvement is very slow and significant improvement in gastric mucosal histology is only observed after many years of follow-up [46, 47]. Failure to achieve complete remission by *H. pylori* eradication in the majority of patients does not necessarily argue against the role of *H. pylori* in the pathogenesis of autoimmune gastritis but, more likely, indicates that a point of no return may be reached beyond which the autoimmune process may no longer require the continued presence of the inducing pathogen.

Recommendations for the Diagnostic Workup of Refractory or Obscure IDA

In view of the above considerations, a rapid screening for celiac disease (anti-endomysial antibodies), autoimmune type A atrophic gastritis (gastrin, anti-parietal antibodies), and *H. pylori* (IgG antibodies followed by urease breath test) may provide a high-sensitivity screening and an effective starting point for further investigations. This is particularly recommended in all patients with obscure IDA and in those refractory to oral iron treatment. The implications of diagnosing celiac disease or autoimmune atrophic gastritis for abnormal iron absorption are obvious. Interpretation of positive serology for *H. pylori* confirmed by positive urease breath test requires clinical judgment as 20–50% of the general and largely healthy population in industrialized countries will have such findings.

In such patients, refractoriness to oral iron treatment may justify a 'test-and-treat' approach of *H. pylori* eradication as recommended by the Maastricht III European Consensus Conference [48, 49]. Cure of previously refractory IDA by *H. pylori* eradication, documented by a negative repeat urease breath test, could then be regarded as evidence supporting a cause-and-effect relation.

References

1 Cook JD, Skikne BS, Baynes RD: Iron deficiency: the global perspective. Adv Exp Med Biol 1994;356:219–228.

2 Rockey DC, Cello JP: Evaluation of the gastrointestinal tract in patients with iron-deficiency anemia. N Engl J Med 1993;329:1691–1695.

3 McIntyre AS, Long RG: Prospective survey of investigations in outpatients referred with iron deficiency anaemia. Gut 1993;34:1102–1107.

4 Bini EJ, Micale PL, Weinshel EH: Evaluation of the gastrointestinal tract in premenopausal women with iron deficiency anemia Am J Med 1998;105:281–286.

5 Dickey W, Hughes D: Prevalence of celiac disease and its endoscopic markers among patients having routine upper gastrointestinal endoscopy. Am J Gastroenterol 1999;94:2182–2186.

6 Choe YH, Kwon YS, Jung MK, Kang SK, Hwang TS, Hong YC: *Helicobacter pylori*-associated iron-deficiency anemia in adolescent female athletes. J Pediatr 2001;139:100–104.

7 Annibale B, Marignani M, Monarca B, Antonelli G, Marcheggiano A, Martino G, Mandelli F, Caprilli R, Delle Fave G: Reversal of iron deficiency anemia after *Helicobacter pylori* eradication in patients with asymptomatic gastritis. Ann Intern Med 1999;131:668–672.

8 Annibale B, Capurso G, Chistolini A, D'Ambra G, DiGiulio E, Monarca B, Delle-Fave G: Gastrointestinal causes of refractory iron deficiency anemia in patients without gastrointestinal symptoms. Am J Med 2001;111:439–445.

9 Dickey W, Kenny BD, McMillan SA, Porter KG, McConnell JB: Gastric as well as duodenal biopsies may be useful in the investigation of iron deficiency anaemia. Scand J Gastroenterol 1997;32:469–472.

10 Halfdanarson TR, Litzow MR, Murray JA: Hematologic manifestations of celiac disease. Blood 2007;109:412–421.

11 Bottaro G, Cataldo F, Rotolo N, Spina M, Corazza GR: The clinical pattern of subclinical/silent celiac disease: an analysis on 1026 consecutive cases. Am J Gastroenterol 1999;94:691–696.

12 Corazza GR, Valentini RA, Andreani ML, D'Anchino M, Leva MT, Ginaldi L, De Feudis L, Quaglino D, Gasbarrini G: Subclinical coeliac disease is a frequent cause of iron-deficiency anaemia. Scand J Gastroenterol 1995;30:153–156.

13 Carroccio A, Iannitto E, Cavataio F, Montalto G, Tumminello M, Campagna P, Lipari MG, Notarbartolo A, Iacono G: Sideropenic anemia and celiac disease: one study, two points of view. Dig Dis Sci 1998;43:673–678.

14 Annibale B, Capurso G, Chistolini A, D'Ambra G, DiGiulio E, Monarca B, Delle-Fave G: Gastrointestinal causes of refractory iron deficiency anemia in patients without gastrointestinal symptoms. Am J Med 2001;111:439–445.

15 Howard MR, Turnbull AJ, Morley P, Hollier P, Webb R, Clarke A: A prospective study of the prevalence of undiagnosed coeliac disease in laboratory defined iron and folate deficiency. J Clin Pathol 2002;55:754–757.

16 Mandal AK, Mehdi I, Munshi SK, Lo TC: Value of routine duodenal biopsy in diagnosing coeliac disease in patients with iron deficiency anaemia. Postgrad Med J 2004;80:475–477.

17 Chorzelski TP, Beutner EH, Sulej J, Tchorzewska H, Jablonska S, Kumar V, Kapuscinska A: IgA anti-endomysium antibody. A new immunological marker of dermatitis herpetiformis and coeliac disease. Br J Dermatol 1984;111:395–402.

18 Faber K: Achylia gastrica mit Anämie. Med Klin 1909;5:1310–1325.

19 Wintrobe MM, Beebe RT: Idiopathic hypochromic anemia. Medicine 1933;12:187–243.

20 Hershko C, Hoffbrand AV, Keret D, Souroujon M, Maschler I, Monselise Y, Lahad A: Role of autoimmune gastritis, *Helicobacter pylori* and celiac disease in refractory or unexplained iron deficiency anemia. Haematologica 2005;90:585–595.

21 Cook JD, Brown GM, Valberg LS: The effect of achylia gastrica on iron absorption. J Clin Invest 1964;43:1185–1191.

22 Schade SG, Cohen RJ, Conrad ME: The effect of hydrochloric acid on iron absorption. N Engl J Med 1968;279:621–624.

23 Bezwoda W, Charlton R, Bothwell T, Torrance J, Mayet F: The importance of gastric hydrochloric acid in the absorption of nonheme food iron. J Lab Clin Med 1978;92:108–116.

24 Milman N, Rosenstock S, Andersen L, Jørgensen T, Bonnevie O: Serum ferritin, hemoglobin, and *Helicobacter pylori* infection: a seroepidemiologic survey comprising 2794 Danish adults. Gastroenterology 1998;115:268–274.

25 Baggett HC, Parkinson AJ, Muth PT, Gold BD, Gessner BD: Endemic iron deficiency associated with *Helicobacter pylori* infection among school-aged children in Alaska. Pediatrics 2006;117:e396–e404.

26 Parkinson AJ, Gold BD, Bulkow L, Wainwright RB, Swaminathan B, Khanna B, Petersen KM, Fitzgerald MA: High prevalence of *Helicobacter pylori* in the Alaska native population and association with low serum ferritin levels in young adults. Clin Diagn Lab Immunol 2000;7:885–888.

27 Cardenas VM, Mulla ZD, Ortiz M, Graham DY: Iron deficiency and *Helicobacter pylori* infection in the United States. Am J Epidemiol 2006;163:127–134.

28 Suerbaum S, Michetti P: *Helicobacter pylori* infection. N Engl J Med 2002;347:1175–1186.

29 Dufour C, Brisigotti M, Fabretti G, Luxardo P, Mori PG, Barabino A: *Helicobacter pylori* gastric infection and sideropenic refractory anemia. J Pediatr Gastroenterol Nutr 1993;17:225–227.

30 Choe YH, Kim SK, Son BK, Lee DH, Hong YC, Pai SH: Randomized placebo-controlled trial of *Helicobacter pylori* eradication for iron-deficiency anemia in preadolescent children and adolescents. Helicobacter 1999;4:135–139.

31 Choe YH, Lee JE, Kim SK: Effect of *Helicobacter pylori* eradication on sideropenic refractory anaemia in adolescent girls with *Helicobacter pylori* infection. Acta Paediatr 2000;89:154–157.

32 Hershko C, Ianculovich M, Souroujon M: A hematologist's view of unexplained iron deficiency anemia in males: impact of *Helicobacter pylori* eradication. Blood Cells Mol Dis 2007;38:45–53.

33 Beutler E: Hepcidin mimetics from microorganisms? A possible explanation for the effect of *Helicobacter pylori* on iron homeostasis (commentary). Blood Cells Mol Dis 2007;38:54–56.

34 Du X, She E, Gelbart T: The serine protease TMPRSS6 is required to sense iron deficiency. Science 2008;320:1088–1092.

35 Ciacci C, Sabbatini F, Cavallaro R, Castiglione F, Di Bella S, Iovino P, Palumbo A, Tortora R, Amoruso D, Mazzacca G: *Helicobacter pylori* impairs iron absorption in infected individuals. Dig Liver Dis 2004;36:455–460.

36 Annibale B, Capurso G, Lahner E, Passi S, Ricci R, Maggio F, Delle Fave G: Concomitant alterations in intragastric pH and ascorbic acid concentration in patients with *Helicobacter pylori* gastritis and associated iron deficiency anaemia. Gut 2003;52:496–501.

37 Hershko C, Ronson A, Souroujon M, Maschler I, Heyd J, Patz J: Variable hematologic presentation of autoimmune gastritis: age-related progression from iron deficiency to cobalamin depletion. Blood 2006;107:1673–1679.

38 Stopeck A: Links between *Helicobacter pylori* infection, cobalamin deficiency, and pernicious anemia. Arch Intern Med 2000;160:1229–1230.

39 Appelmelk BJ, Simoons-Smit I, Negrini R, Moran AP, Aspinall GO, Forte JG, De Vries T, Quan H, Verboom T, Maaskant JJ, Ghiara P, Kuipers EJ, Bloemena E, Tadema TM, Townsend RR, Tyagarajan K, Crothers JM Jr, Monteiro MA, Savio A, De Graaff J: Potential role of molecular mimicry between *Helicobacter pylori* lipopolysaccharide and host Lewis blood group antigens in autoimmunity. Infect Immun 1996;64:2031–2040.

40 Claeys D, Faller G, Appelmelk BJ, Negrini R, Kirchner T: The gastric H+,K+-ATPase is a major autoantigen in chronic *Helicobacter pylori* gastritis with body mucosa atrophy. Gastroenterology 1998;115:340–347.

41 Negrini R, Savio A, Poiesi C, Appelmelk BJ, Buffoli F, Paterlini A, Cesari P, Graffeo M, Vaira D, Franzin G: Antigenic mimicry between *Helicobacter pylori* and gastric mucosa in the pathogenesis of body atrophic gastritis. Gastroenterology 1996;111:655–665.

42 Rad R, Schmid RM, Prinz C: *Helicobacter pylori*, iron deficiency, and gastric autoimmunity. Blood 2006;107:4969–4970.

43 Annibale B, Di Giulio E, Caruana P, Lahner E, Capurso G, Bordi C, Delle Fave G: The long-term effects of cure of *Helicobacter pylori* infection on patients with atrophic body gastritis. Aliment Pharmacol Ther 2002;16:1723–1731.

44 Kaptan K, Beyan C, Ural AU, Cetin T, Avcu F, Gülşen M, Finci R, Yalçín A: *Helicobacter pylori* – is it a novel causative agent in vitamin B$_{12}$ deficiency? Arch Intern Med 2000;160:1349–1353.

45 Haruma K, Mihara M, Okamoto E, Kusunoki H, Hananoki M, Tanaka S, Yoshihara M, Sumii K, Kajiyama G: Eradication of *Helicobacter pylori* increases gastric acidity in patients with atrophic gastritis of the corpus – evaluation of 24-h pH monitoring. Aliment Pharmacol Ther 1999;13:155–162.

46 You WC, Brown LM, Zhang L, Li JY, Jin ML, Chang YS, Ma JL, Pan KF, Liu WD, Hu Y, Crystal-Mansour S, Pee D, Blot WJ, Fraumeni JF Jr, Xu GW, Gail MH: Randomized double-blind factorial trial of three treatments to reduce the prevalence of precancerous gastric lesions. J Natl Cancer Inst 2006;98:974–983.

47 Mera R, Fontham ET, Bravo LE, Bravo JC, Piazuelo MB, Camargo MC, Correa P: Re: long term follow up of patients treated for *Helicobacter pylori* infection. Gut 2005;54:1536–1540.

48 Bourke B, Ceponis P, Chiba N, Czinn S, Ferraro R, Fischbach L, Gold B, Hyunh H, Jacobson K, Jones NL, Koletzko S, Lebel S, Moayyedi P, Ridell R, Sherman P, van Zanten S, Beck I, Best L, Boland M, Bursey F, Chaun H, Cooper G, Craig B, Creuzenet C, Critch J, Govender K, Hassall E, Kaplan A, Keelan M, Noad G, Robertson M, Smith L, Stein M, Taylor D, Walters T, Persaud R, Whitaker S, Woodland R, Canadian Helicobacter Study Group: Canadian Helicobacter Study Group Consensus Conference: update on the approach to *Helicobacter pylori* infection in children and adolescents – an evidence-based evaluation. Can J Gastroenterol 2005;19:399–408.

49 Malfertheiner P, Megraud F, O'Morain C, Bazzoli F, El-Omar E, Graham D, Hunt R, Rokkas T, Vakil N, Kuipers EJ: Current concepts in the management of *Helicobacter pylori* infection: the Maastricht III Consensus Report. Gut 2007;56:772–781.

50 Hershko C, Ronson A, Souroujon M, Cabantchik ZI, Patz J: Mechanisms of iron regulation and of iron deficiency. Haematol Hematol Edu 2007;1:1–9.

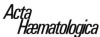

Acta Haematol 2009;122:103–108
DOI: 10.1159/000243794

Published online: November 10, 2009

Anemia of Chronic Disease (Anemia of Inflammation)

Neeraj Agarwal[a]   Josef T. Prchal[a, b]

[a]Division of Hematology and Oncology, University of Utah School of Medicine and Veterans Affairs Hospital, and
[b]ARUP Laboratories, Salt Lake City, Utah, USA

Key Words

Chronic disease · Erythropoietin · Hepcidin · Hypoferremia · Inflammation · Transferrin

Abstract

Mild-to-moderate anemia often develops in the setting of acute or chronic immune activation and is termed anemia of chronic disease (ACD) or anemia of inflammation. Anemia of chronic disease is the second most common type of anemia (after anemia of iron deficiency) and results in increased morbidity and mortality of the underlying disease. Anemia of chronic disease is mediated by inflammatory cytokines and is characterized by low serum iron (hypoferremia) and often increased reticuloendothelial stores of iron. Hepcidin is the master regulator of iron homeostasis and its synthesis is inhibited by iron deficiency and stimulated by inflammation. The serum hepcidin level is useful in identifying iron deficiency in patients with ACD. Successful treatment of the underlying disease improves ACD. If that is not possible and if anemia is symptomatic, treatment with erythropoietic agents, supplemented with iron if necessary, is helpful in many cases.

Copyright © 2009 S. Karger AG, Basel

Definition

Mild-to-moderate anemia often develops in the setting of chronic disease, infections or malignancy, and is known as anemia of chronic disease (ACD) [1]. Because the underlying cause of ACD is an acute or a chronic activation of immune response, a more specific term is anemia of inflammation [2]. Anemia of inflammation is one of the most common causes of anemia, along with anemia of iron deficiency.

Pathophysiology

Multiple factors have been shown to be associated with the pathogenesis of mild-to-moderate anemia seen in the setting of chronic disease. The most important of these is iron-limited erythropoiesis, which is mediated by increased levels of serum hepcidin.

Iron Homeostasis

Iron metabolism has been reviewed by Nemeth and Ganz in this issue [pp 78–86] and is therefore only briefly described here. Although the average male has 1–2 g of iron stores, normally only 1–2 mg is lost daily (through the shedding of intestinal mucosal cells) and 1–2 mg is absorbed daily through the gut [3]. Far more iron is generated from senescent erythrocytes and ~20 mg of iron is recycled by macrophages every day. Dietary iron is absorbed from the intestinal lumen into the duodenal enterocytes by a divalent metal transporter protein, known as DMT1. DMT1 is highly expressed at the brush border of the apical pole of the enterocytes in the proximal duodenum, and also plays also a crucial role in utilizing iron released from transferrin in the endosomes of erythroblasts for effective erythropoiesis [4]. Ferroportin is the

Prof. Josef T. Prchal, MD
Division of Hematology
30 North 1900 East, SOM 5C402
Salt Lake City, UT 84132 (USA)
Tel. +1 801 581 4220, Fax +1 801 585 3432, E-Mail josef.prchal@hsc.utah.edu

major iron exporter protein and is found on the basolateral surface of duodenal enterocytes, macrophages, and hepatocytes. Once absorbed into the duodenal enterocytes, ferroportin exports iron into the circulation. In circulation, iron is carried by transferrin (each molecule can carry two atoms of iron in ferric form), which delivers the iron to erythrocyte precursors in the marrow to be incorporated into hemoglobin (Hb). Senescent erythrocytes are phagocytosed by the macrophages, which store iron as ferritin. Each ferritin molecule can store up to 4,500 atoms of iron within its spherical cavity [5]. As needed, macrophages export iron via ferroportin to transferrin, making iron available for erythropoiesis and all other cells. Iron homeostasis is regulated by hepcidin, a bactericidal peptide hormone made by hepatocytes [3].

Hepcidin and Iron Homeostasis

Hepcidin is a 25-amino-acid peptide hormone which is synthesized in hepatocytes, circulates in the plasma, and is excreted in the urine. Hepcidin controls the release of iron from macrophages by its action on the iron exporter protein, ferroportin. Upon binding with hepcidin, ferroportin molecules dissociate from the membrane and become internalized, phosphorylated, and degraded [6, 7]. This leads to a diminished release of iron from macrophage stores, as well as a diminished export of iron from duodenal enterocytes, resulting in decreased serum iron. In the presence of chronic inflammation, the persistent elevation in serum hepcidin results in a gradual accumulation of iron in the macrophages as they continue to phagocytose older erythrocytes, but do not release this iron for ongoing erythropoiesis. This, together with a diminished absorption of iron from the duodenum, leads to ACD.

Regulation of Hepcidin Level

Hepcidin, encoded by the *Hamp* gene, is regulated at the transcriptional and posttranscriptional levels by multiple extracellular signals. Hepcidin production is upregulated by the inflammatory cytokine interleukin (IL)-6 and lipopolysaccharides [8]. Other factors, which upregulate hepcidin levels, are increased body iron levels, hemochromatosis protein HFE, the transcription factor SMAD4, and bone morphogenetic protein (BMP) [9]. BMP signaling requires hemojuvelin as a coreceptor, and hemojuvelin mutation is associated with hemochromatosis due to impaired BMP signaling [10]. Factors which downregulate hepcidin production include hyperactive erythropoiesis, iron deficiency, anemia, hypoxia, and erythropoietin (EPO) [9]. A potent inhibitor of hepcidin

is TMPRSS6, which encodes a type II transmembrane serine protease produced by the liver. The TMPRSS6-dependent pathway predominates over all known *Hamp*-activating pathways, since the overexpression of TMPRSS6 partially or fully nullifies the hepcidin-inducing effects of hemojuvelin, BMP2, BMP4, BMP9, SMAD1, IL-1, and IL-6. Germline mutations in TMPRSS6 result in iron deficiency anemia (IDA), which is refractory to oral iron therapy but improves with parenteral iron therapy [11, 12].

Erythropoiesis directly downregulates hepcidin production and increases iron absorption [9]. During increased (although ineffective) erythropoiesis in thalassemia intermedia or major, a high level of a cytokine growth differentiation factor 15 (GDF15) inhibits hepcidin expression, contributing to both an increase in iron absorption and iron overload, characteristic of thalassemia [13]. Recently, another erythroid suppressor of hepcidin expression, named twisted gastrulation (TWSG1) was demonstrated to interfere with BMP-mediated hepcidin expression [14].

Other Factors Involved in the Pathogenesis of ACD

These include suboptimal EPO activity (either due to diminished EPO production or resistance, or both), decreased erythrocyte life span, and an inhibitory effect of cytokines on erythroid progenitors.

EPO gene expression is inhibited by the inflammatory cytokines IL-1 and tumor necrosis factor (TNF) in vitro and by lipopolysaccharides in mice [15]. Inflammatory cytokines increase the binding activity of the transcription factor GATA and inhibit EPO gene promoter activity. GATA-1 inhibitor negates this inhibitory effect of inflammatory cytokines and increases EPO transcription [16]. Interferon (IFN)-γ or TNF-α reduces the sensitivity of erythroid progenitor cells to EPO and, subsequently, higher levels of EPO are required to restore the formation of human erythroid colony-forming units [17]. This is partly due to cytokine-associated downregulation of EPO receptors on erythroid progenitor cells [2]. In addition, the proinflammatory cytokines TNF-α and IL-1β inhibit transferrin receptor (TfR) expression and TNF-α and IFN-γ enhance ferritin H-chain expression in vitro [18].

The survival of erythrocytes from patients with anemia of inflammation when transfused into normal individuals is not diminished. However, the survival of erythrocytes from a normal individual transfused to individuals with chronic disease is decreased [1]. This suggests factors extrinsic to erythrocytes cause decreased red cell

Table 1. Laboratory evaluation of ACD, IDA and a combination of both

Laboratory parameters	ACD	IDA	ACD/IDA
Serum iron	↓	↓	↓
Transferrin (TIBC)	↓	↑	↓ or ↑
Ferritin	↑	↓	↑ or ↓ (only in case of severe iron deficiency)
sTfR	↓ or N	↑	↑ or ↓
sTfR-F index	0.8 (median)	5.4 (median)	3.2 (median)
Serum hepcidin	↑	↓	↓
Marrow iron	↑ (only in macrophages)	↓	↓

N = Normal; ↓ = reduced; ↑ = increased; TIBC = total iron binding capacity.

survival in the environment of inflammation [19]. IFN-γ and TNF-α induce nitric oxide synthase and generate nitric oxide, which inhibits erythropoiesis in a dose-dependent fashion. However, the pathophysiology of anemia of inflammation is not fully elucidated, as suggested by the related condition, 'anemia of aging', wherein anemia is not associated with increased hepcidin [20, 21].

Laboratory Findings

Hb Level and Erythrocyte Morphology

Hb levels are mildly (10–11 g/dl) to moderately decreased (8–9 g/dl). Erythrocytes are usually normocytic and normochromic. However, with more severe anemia, erythrocytes can become hypochromic and microcytic [1].

Serum Iron Studies

Serum iron is typically low. The serum transferrin concentration (also defined as iron-binding capacity) is decreased or low-normal. Because of the concomitant decline in serum iron as well as serum transferrin concentration, serum transferrin saturation may be normal. In contrast, in IDA, serum iron is low, but serum transferrin is high, which results in low serum transferrin saturation (summarized in table 1). Serum ferritin is an acute-phase protein and its level increases in ACD as a result of inflammation and increased iron stores. IDA, in contrast, has a low serum ferritin concentration. In ACD, a serum ferritin concentration <60 ng/ml is suggestive of concomitant iron deficiency [22]. In a study of patients with ACD, all patients with serum ferritin levels <30 ng/ml had iron deficiency by marrow examination. However, in this study, one third of the patients with serum ferritin between 100

and 200 ng/ml also had iron deficiency, suggesting a low specificity of serum iron, transferrin, and ferritin as diagnostic measures of anemia of inflammation [23].

Soluble TfR

A useful measure of iron deficiency is soluble TfR (sTfR). TfR is a transmembrane protein which binds iron-containing transferrin. TfR is present on virtually all cells in the body, but is found at high concentrations on Hb-synthesizing erythroid precursors. An increased iron requirement, as well as hyperactive erythropoiesis, increases the synthesis of TfR. These receptors bind to iron-carrying serum transferrin molecules and form TfR-transferrin-iron complexes. These complexes are internalized by endocytosis and transported to the cytoplasm where they fuse with endosomes. In the acidic atmosphere of endosomes, iron is released from transferrin and the apotransferrin-TfR complex is recycled to the cell surface where, at neutral pH, apotransferrin is released to enter the circulation. Iron is then transported by DMT1 from endosomes and is available in mitochondria for Hb synthesis. This complex, yet not fully elucidated process has been the subject of several recent reviews [24, 25]. In plasma, sTfR is a truncated form of the tissue receptor, and its serum concentration is directly proportional to the iron requirement in the cells [26].

sTfR/log Ferritin Ratio (TfR-F Index)

Because of the unreliable nature of serum ferritin in the presence of inflammation and increased TfR synthesis from augmented erythropoiesis that is independent of iron deficiency, a ratio of sTfR/log ferritin has been proposed to be useful in predicting iron deficiency in patients with ACD [27]. In a study of 129 consecutive anemic patients, all of whom underwent marrow examination, 48 had IDA, 64 had ACD and 17 had a combination of ACD and IDA (ACD/IDA) [28]. Serum TfR concentrations were elevated in most patients with IDA and patients with ACD/IDA, but not in patients with ACD alone. Calculation of the TfR-F index did not considerably improve diagnostic efficiency compared with TfR alone. However, logarithmic transformation of ferritin values and calculation of the TfR-F index provided a reliable indicator of iron depletion and correlated with the bone marrow findings. The median values of TfR-F indices for each patient group were 5.4 for IDA, 3.2 for ACD/IDA and 0.8 for ACD.

Serum Hepcidin Concentration

Hepcidin is the master regulator of iron homeostasis and its synthesis is inhibited by iron deficiency and stimulated by inflammation. The serum hepcidin level has the potential to identify iron deficiency in patients with ACD. However, a reliable assay to measure serum hepcidin was not available until recently, when a serum enzyme-linked immunosorbent assay for serum hepcidin was reported [29]. In this study of healthy volunteers, the median serum hepcidin concentrations were 112 ng/ml (range 29–254) in men and 65 ng/ml (range 17–286) in women. Serum hepcidin levels were also tested in patients with a variety of clinical conditions associated with iron disturbances. Serum hepcidin concentrations were undetectable or low in patients with IDA (ferritin <10 ng/ml), iron-depleted HFE hemochromatosis, and juvenile hemochromatosis. Serum hepcidin concentrations were high in patients with inflammation (C-reactive protein >10 mg/dl), multiple myeloma, or chronic kidney disease. More recently, serum hepcidin concentrations were assessed in patients with ACD, IDA or both diseases [30]. Serum hepcidin levels were significantly decreased in patients with IDA and ACD/IDA and elevated in ACD compared with controls. Notably, there was no difference between serum IL-6 levels in subjects with ACD (with high serum hepcidin) and ACD/IDA subjects (with low serum hepcidin) [30]. This report suggests that the erythroid demand for iron is a more powerful regulator of hepcidin expression than inflammation. Because of clearly different levels of serum hepcidin in subjects with ACD and ACD/IDA in this study, estimation of serum hepcidin is considered a valuable tool to assess iron deficiency in subjects with ACD [30].

Bone Marrow Examination

The marrow iron is considered the gold standard for the diagnosis of iron deficiency. In subjects with IDA, marrow iron stores are depleted in both erythroid progenitors as well as macrophages. However, in ACD, iron stains show increased iron in macrophages, but iron is decreased/absent in erythroid precursors.

Treatment

Treatment of the underlying disease usually alleviates ACD. However, no treatment of anemia is needed if it is mild and asymptomatic. In symptomatic patients with more severe anemia, erythropoiesis-stimulating agents can be used to improve the Hb level. Currently, the following three different recombinant human EPOs (rhEPO) are commonly used: epoetin-α (Procrit; Johnson & Johnson, New Brunswick, N.J., and Epogen; Amgen, Thousand Oaks, Calif., USA), epoetin-β (Recormon; Roche Diagnostics, Basel, Switzerland), and a second-generation erythropoietic agent, darbepoetin-α (Aranesp; Amgen). Native EPO has a half-life of 8.5 h. After subcutaneous injection, the half-lives of rhEPOs in plasma increase in the following manner: epoetin-α to 20.5 h, epoetin-β to 24 h, and darbepoetin-α to 49 h. Despite different pharmacodynamic and pharmacokinetic properties, all these products are considered to have similar clinical efficacy [31, 32]. However, these agents are not approved by the United States Food and Drug Administration (FDA) to treat all types of ACD. Currently, Epogen, Procrit and Aranesp are approved by the FDA to treat anemia in patients with chronic kidney failure and anemia caused by chemotherapy in certain patients with cancer. Epogen and Procrit are also approved for use in certain patients with anemia who are scheduled to undergo major surgery to reduce blood transfusions during or shortly after surgery and for the treatment of anemia associated with zidovudine (AZT) therapy in HIV patients [33]. Continuous EPO receptor activator (Mircera, Hoffmann-La Roche, Nutley, N.J., USA) is another FDA-approved rhEPO which is longer acting and needs to be administered only once every month. It is composed of a large methoxy-polyethylene glycol polymer chain integrated into the EPO molecule and linked primarily by amide bonds, resulting in a longer half-life (~130 h after both intravenous and subcutaneous administration) [34]. Mircera was shown to be efficacious in the management of anemia of chronic renal disease when given intravenously at 2- or 4-week dosing intervals [35, 36]. It is currently in clinical use in England but not in the United States.

For epoetin-α and -β, the recommended dosing is as follows: administered subcutaneously, 150 units/kg 3 times/week or 10,000 units 3 times/week or 40,000 units once weekly, to achieve and maintain Hb levels between 10 and 12 g/dl. For darbepoetin, the recommended dosing is as follows: administered subcutaneously, 2.25 μg/kg once weekly or 200 μg every 2 weeks or 500 μg once every 3 weeks, to achieve and maintain Hb levels between 10–12 g/dl. EPO supplementation should not be started if the Hb level is ≥10 g/dl. Hb levels should not exceed 12 g/dl and should not rise >1 g/dl per 2-week time period during therapy in any patient. EPO supplementation should be discontinued if suboptimal or no response (i.e. <1–2 g/dl rise in Hb) is evident after 6–8 weeks of use [37].

One of the reasons for failure of EPO supplementation to improve ACD is concomitant iron deficiency. Iron deficiency in a patient with ACD is indicated by one or more of the following factors: low ferritin (<60 ng/ml), low transferrin saturation (<20%), TfR-F >3.2, very low or undetectable serum hepcidin concentration, or diminished stainable iron in the marrow. Oral iron replacement is usually adequate for most patients. However, parenteral iron supplementation may be necessary in the presence of one or more of the following: unreliable absorption through the gut (due to underlying disease), intolerance or resistance to oral iron supplementation, and relatively severe or symptomatic anemia [38]. Although iron supplementation may not correct anemia, it should be continued until iron deficiency has been corrected, as evidenced by improvement in the above-mentioned markers of iron deficiency.

Functional EPO receptors have been identified in non-erythroid cells, including endothelial, muscle, and neural cells. There is increasing evidence that EPO can act to stimulate cell proliferation and cell-specific function, or promote cell survival in these tissues [39]. Several clinical trials of patients with different cancers have demonstrated an increased risk of venous thromboembolism, as well as worsening of survival with EPO treatment [40–42]. Many of these patients received intravenous iron supplementation; iron stimulates tumor growth, while iron chelation retards tumor growth and stimulates rapid ubiquitination and proteasomal destruction of cyclin D and other cancer-promoting cell cycle regulators [43, 44]. However, EPO treatment of anemia in chronic heart failure patients may not be associated with increased morbidity and mortality [please also see the review by Silverberg et al. in this issue, pp 109–119]. In a recent meta-analysis, EPO supplementation in patients with chronic heart failure was not associated with a higher mortality rate or more adverse events, but beneficially affected hospitalization for heart failure [45]. Strict adherence to guidelines when using EPO to treat ACD should be followed, and use of EPO should be discontinued if suboptimal or no benefit is observed within 6–8 weeks.

References

1 Cartwright GE: The anemia of chronic disorders. Semin Hematol 1966;3:351–375.
2 Weiss G, Goodnough LT: Anemia of chronic disease. N Engl J Med 2005;352:1011–1023.
3 Ganz T, Nemeth E: Regulation of iron acquisition and iron distribution in mammals. Biochim Biophys Acta 2006;1763:690–699.
4 Mims MP, Guan Y, Pospisilova D, Priwitzerova M, Indrak K, Ponka P, Divoky V, Prchal JT: Identification of a human mutation of DMT1 in a patient with microcytic anemia and iron overload. Blood 2005;105:1337–1342.
5 Harrison PM, Arosio P: The ferritins: molecular properties, iron storage function and cellular regulation. Biochim Biophys Acta 1996;1275:161–203.
6 Nemeth E, Tuttle MS, Powelson J, Vaughn MB, Donovan A, Ward DM, Ganz T, Kaplan J: Hepcidin regulates cellular iron efflux by binding to ferroportin and inducing its internalization. Science 2004;306:2090–2093.

7 De Domenico I, Lo E, Ward DM, Kaplan J: Hepcidin-induced internalization of ferroportin requires binding and cooperative interaction with Jak2. Proc Natl Acad Sci USA 2009;106:3800–3805.
8 Nemeth E, Valore EV, Territo M, Schiller G, Lichtenstein A, Ganz T: Hepcidin, a putative mediator of anemia of inflammation, is a type II acute-phase protein. Blood 2003;101:2461–2463.
9 Nemeth E: Iron regulation and erythropoiesis. Curr Opin Hematol 2008;15:169–175.
10 Babitt JL, Huang FW, Wrighting DM, Xia Y, Sidis Y, Samad TA, Campagna JA, Chung RT, Schneyer AL, Woolf CJ, Andrews NC, Lin HY: Bone morphogenetic protein signaling by hemojuvelin regulates hepcidin expression. Nat Genet 2006;38:531–539.
11 Du X, She E, Gelbart T, Truksa J, Lee P, Xia Y, Khovananth K, Mudd S, Mann N, Moresco EM, Beutler E, Beutler B: The serine protease TMPRSS6 is required to sense iron deficiency. Science 2008;320:1088–1092.

12 Truksa J, Lee P, Beutler E: Two BMP responsive elements, STAT, and bZIP/HNF4/COUP motifs of the hepcidin promoter are critical for BMP, SMAD1, and HJV responsiveness. Blood 2009;113:688–695.
13 Tanno T, Bhanu NV, Oneal PA, Goh SH, Staker P, Lee YT, Moroney JW, Reed CH, Luban NL, Wang RH, Eling TE, Childs R, Ganz T, Leitman SF, Fucharoen S, Miller JL: High levels of GDF15 in thalassemia suppress expression of the iron regulatory protein hepcidin. Nat Med 2007;13:1096–1101.
14 Tanno T, Porayette P, Sripichai O, Noh SJ, Byrnes C, Bhupatiraju A, Lee YT, Goodnough JB, Harandi O, Ganz T, Paulson RF, Miller JL: Identification of TWSG1 as a second novel erythroid regulator of hepcidin expression in murine and human cells. Blood 2009;114:181–186.
15 Jelkmann W: Proinflammatory cytokines lowering erythropoietin production. J Interferon Cytokine Res 1998;18:555–559.

16 Imagawa S, Nakano Y, Obara N, Suzuki N, Doi T, Kodama T, Nagasawa T, Yamamoto M: A GATA-specific inhibitor (K-7174) rescues anemia induced by IL-1β, TNF-α, or L-NMMA. FASEB J 2003;17:1742–1744.

17 Means RT Jr, Krantz SB: Inhibition of human erythroid colony-forming units by gamma interferon can be corrected by recombinant human erythropoietin. Blood 1991;78:2564–2567.

18 Fahmy M, Young SP: Modulation of iron metabolism in monocyte cell line U937 by inflammatory cytokines: changes in transferrin uptake, iron handling and ferritin mRNA. Biochem J 1993;296:175–181.

19 Means RT Jr: Recent developments in the anemia of chronic disease. Curr Hematol Rep 2003;2:116–121.

20 Maciejewski JP, Selleri C, Sato T, Cho HJ, Keefer LK, Nathan CF, Young NS: Nitric oxide suppression of human hematopoiesis in vitro. Contribution to inhibitory action of interferon-gamma and tumor necrosis factor-alpha. J Clin Invest 1995;96:1085–1092.

21 Lee P, Gelbart T, Waalen J, Beutler E: The anemia of ageing is not associated with increased plasma hepcidin levels. Blood Cells Mol Dis 2008;41:252–254.

22 Witte DL: Can serum ferritin be effectively interpreted in the presence of the acute-phase response? Clin Chem 1991;37:484–485.

23 North M, Dallalio G, Donath AS, Melink R, Means RT Jr: Serum transferrin receptor levels in patients undergoing evaluation of iron stores: correlation with other parameters and observed versus predicted results. Clin Lab Haematol 1997;19:93–97.

24 Lee PL, Beutler E: Regulation of hepcidin and iron-overload disease. Annu Rev Pathol 2009;4:489–515.

25 Zhang AS, Enns CA: Iron homeostasis: recently identified proteins provide insight into novel control mechanisms. J Biol Chem 2009;284:711–715.

26 Cook JD, Skikne BS, Baynes RD: Serum transferrin receptor. Annu Rev Med 1993;44:63–74.

27 Skikne BS, Flowers CH, Cook JD: Serum transferrin receptor: a quantitative measure of tissue iron deficiency. Blood 1990;75:1870–1876.

28 Punnonen K, Irjala K, Rajamaki A: Serum transferrin receptor and its ratio to serum ferritin in the diagnosis of iron deficiency. Blood 1997;89:1052–1057.

29 Ganz T, Olbina G, Girelli D, Nemeth E, Westerman M: Immunoassay for human serum hepcidin. Blood 2008;112:4292–4297.

30 Theurl I, Aigner E, Theurl M, Nairz M, Seifert M, Schroll A, Sonnweber T, Eberwein L, Witcher DR, Murphy AT, Wroblewski VJ, Wurz E, Datz C, Weiss G: Regulation of iron homeostasis in anemia of chronic disease and iron deficiency anemia: diagnostic and therapeutic implications. Blood 2009;113:5277–5286.

31 Egrie JC, Dwyer E, Browne JK, Hitz A, Lykos MA: Darbepoetin alfa has a longer circulating half-life and greater in vivo potency than recombinant human erythropoietin. Exp Hematol 2003;31:290–299.

32 Beutel G, Ganser A: Risks and benefits of erythropoiesis-stimulating agents in cancer management. Semin Hematol 2007;44:157–165.

33 (FDA) US Food and Drug Administration: http://www.fda.gov/bbs/topics/news/2007/new01740.html.

34 Macdougall IC: CERA (continuous erythropoietin receptor activator): a new erythropoiesis-stimulating agent for the treatment of anemia. Curr Hematol Rep 2005;4:436–440.

35 Sulowicz W, Locatelli F, Ryckelynck JP, Balla J, Csiky B, Harris K, Ehrhard P, Beyer U: Once-monthly subcutaneous C.E.R.A. maintains stable hemoglobin control in patients with chronic kidney disease on dialysis and converted directly from epoetin one to three times weekly. Clin J Am Soc Nephrol 2007;2:637–646.

36 Levin NW, Fishbane S, Canedo FV, Zeig S, Nassar GM, Moran JE, Villa G, Beyer U, Oguey D: Intravenous methoxy polyethylene glycol-epoetin beta for haemoglobin control in patients with chronic kidney disease who are on dialysis: a randomised non-inferiority trial (MAXIMA). Lancet 2007;370:1415–1421.

37 National Comprehensive Cancer Network®: NCCN Clinical Practice Guidelines in Oncology™: Cancer- and Chemotherapy-Induced Anemia, version 2.2009. http://www.nccn.org/professionals/physician_gls/pdf/anemia.pdf

38 Silverstein SB, Rodgers GM: Parenteral iron therapy options. Am J Hematol 2004;76:74–78.

39 Chen ZY, Asavaritikrai P, Prchal JT, Noguchi CT: Endogenous erythropoietin signaling is required for normal neural progenitor cell proliferation. J Biol Chem 2007;282:25875–25883.

40 Blau CA: Erythropoietin in cancer: presumption of innocence? Stem Cells 2007;25:2094–2097.

41 Bennett CL, Silver SM, Djulbegovic B, Samaras AT, Blau CA, Gleason KJ, Barnato SE, Elverman KM, Courtney DM, McKoy JM, Edwards BJ, Tigue CC, Raisch DW, Yarnold PR, Dorr DA, Kuzel TM, Tallman MS, Trifilio SM, West DP, Lai SY, Henke M: Venous thromboembolism and mortality associated with recombinant erythropoietin and darbepoetin administration for the treatment of cancer-associated anemia. JAMA 2008;299:914–924.

42 Bohlius J, Schmidlin K, Brillant C, Schwarzer G, Trelle S, Seidenfeld J, Zwahlen M, Clarke M, Weingart O, Kluge S, Piper M, Rades D, Steensma DP, Djulbegovic B, Fey MF, Ray-Coquard I, Machtay M, Moebus V, Thomas G, Untch M, Schumacher M, Egger M, Engert A: Recombinant human erythropoiesis-stimulating agents and mortality in patients with cancer: a meta-analysis of randomised trials. Lancet 2009;373:1532–1542.

43 Necas E, Prchal JT: The diverse functions of lipocalin: a recently-recognized mediator of transferrin independent iron transport, innate immunity, and cancer signaling. Hematologist 2006;3:3.

44 Whitnall M, Howard J, Ponka P, Richardson DR: A class of iron chelators with a wide spectrum of potent antitumor activity that overcomes resistance to chemotherapeutics. Proc Natl Acad Sci USA 2006;103:14901–14906.

45 van der Meer P, Groenveld H, Januzzi JL, van Veldhuisen DJ: Erythropoietin treatment in patients with chronic heart failure: a meta-analysis. Heart 2009;95:1309–1314.

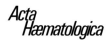

Acta Haematol 2009;122:109–119
DOI: 10.1159/000243795

Published online: November 10, 2009

The Anemia of Heart Failure

Donald S. Silverberg[a]   Dov Wexler[b]   Alberto Palazzuoli[c]   Adrian Iaina[a]
Doron Schwartz[a]

Departments of [a]Nephrology and [b]Cardiology and Heart Failure, Tel Aviv Medical Center, Tel Aviv, Israel;
[c]Section of Cardiology, Department of Internal Medicine and Metabolic Diseases, Le Scotte Hospital,
University of Siena, Siena, Italy

Key Words
Anemia · Chronic kidney disease · Congestive heart failure ·
Dialysis · Erythropoietin · Iron · Renal failure

Abstract
Anemia is common in congestive heart failure (CHF) and is
associated with an increased mortality and morbidity. The
most likely causes of anemia are chronic kidney disease
(CKD) and excessive cytokine production, both of which can
cause depression of erythropoietin (EPO) production and
bone marrow activity. The cytokines also induce iron deficiency by both reducing gastrointestinal iron absorption
and iron release from iron stores located in the macrophages
and hepatocytes. Iron deficiency can cause thrombocytosis
which might also contribute to cardiovascular complications
in both CHF and CKD and is partially reversible with iron
treatment. Thus attempts to control this anemia will have to
consider both the use of erythropoiesis-stimulating agents
(ESA), such as EPO, as well as oral and, probably more importantly, intravenous (IV) iron. The many studies on anemia in
CHF patients treated with ESA and oral or IV iron, and even
with IV iron without ESA have up to now shown a quite consistent positive effect on hospitalization, fatigue, shortness
of breath, quality of life, exercise capacity, and β-natriuretic
peptide reduction, in the absence of increased cardiovascular damage related to the therapy. Adequately powered
long-term placebo-controlled studies of ESA and/or IV iron
are currently being carried out and their results are eagerly
awaited.
Copyright © 2009 S. Karger AG, Basel

Introduction

There are many questions about anemia in congestive heart failure (CHF) which will be dealt with in this
paper. Is anemia common in CHF? How common? Why
is anemia increasing in prevalence in CHF? Is anemia
an independent risk factor for mortality, morbidity, and
hospitalization in CHF? What are the major causes of
anemia in CHF? Is iron deficiency common in CHF?
What causes the iron deficiency? How is iron deficiency
diagnosed in CHF? Does iron treatment improve the
anemia and the general condition of CHF patients? Is
oral iron better than intravenous (IV) iron in chronic
kidney disease (CKD) and in CHF? Is it worthwhile
treating the iron deficiency even if anemia is not present? Does correction of the anemia with erythropoiesis-
stimulating agents (ESA) improve CHF? What is the

Donald S. Silverberg, MD
Department of Nephrology, Tel Aviv Medical Center
Weizman 6
IL–64239 Tel Aviv (Israel)
Tel. +972 9 866 6013, Fax +972 3 546 9825, E-Mail donald@netvision.net.il

target hemoglobin (Hb) in CHF? Are there dangers to the use of ESA and IV iron in CHF? What effect does iron deficiency have on platelet number and function? What effect does an increase in platelets have on inflammation, thrombosis, and atherosclerosis? What are the advantages of using ESA and IV iron alone or in combination in CHF, CKD and the anemia of cancer chemotherapy?

Prevalence and Significance of CHF

Despite the progress made in CHF, mortality and morbidity are still high [1, 2]. In a study by the American Heart Association, in 2006, CHF was mentioned in the death certificates of 292,214 patients [1], and indeed 1 in 8 deaths in the US has CHF mentioned on the death certificate. A CHF diagnosis suggests a poor outcome: the 1-year mortality in patients with a CHF diagnosis amounts to 20%. Hospital discharges for CHF increased from 877,000 in 1996 to 1,106,000 in 2006. The estimated direct and indirect costs of CHF in the US in 2009 are 37.2 billion USD. CHF also continues to be a fatal disease with only 25% surviving 5 years after the first diagnosis [1]. In individuals aged 40, almost 1 in 5 in the US will develop CHF during their remaining life span [1] and, in a Dutch study [2] in individuals aged 55, almost 1 in 3 will develop CHF during their remaining life span.

Prevalence and Significance of Anemia in CHF

Anemia, however it is defined [3], is common in CHF [4–12]. It is found in 30–50% of cases, and is an independent risk factor for more severe CHF, hospitalization and death [4–12]. In addition, the incidence and prevalence of anemia is rising [11, 12]. If defined according to the World Health Organization (WHO) criteria as an Hb concentration <13 g/dl in adult men and <12 g/dl in adult women, it has reached 53% in a recent prospective study of CHF in a community in the US [12]. Is it possible that the anemia may be contributing to the worsening of CHF? In a recent meta-analysis of 34 CHF studies including a total of 153,180 patients, 37.2% were anemic (using the authors' own criteria) and the adjusted hazard ratio for death was 1.46 in these anemic CHF patients [10]. Most anemic CHF patients also have moderate-to-severe CKD as judged by a glomerular filtration rate < 60 ml/min/1.73 m^2 [4–12]. This combination of anemia, CKD and

CHF has been called the cardio-renal anemia syndrome [4, 7] by the authors. The three conditions appear to interact, each one causing or worsening the other two. Thus adequate treatment of all three might prevent the progression of both CKD and CHF.

What Causes the Anemia in CHF?

Anemia associated with CHF is likely due to a combination of several factors [2–7, 11, 12]

Chronic Kidney Disease
CKD is associated with reduced production of erythropoietin (EPO) in the kidney. The renal damage seen in CHF is probably mainly due to reduced renal blood flow caused by the reduced cardiac output causing hypoxic renal damage. Indeed, both anemia and CHF are strong independent risk factors for progression of renal disease [13].

Elevated Cytokines
These are elaborated in CHF, especially tumor necrosis factor (TNF)-α and interleukin (IL)-6. They can cause four hematological abnormalities [14, 15]:

(i) reduced EPO production in the kidney leading to inappropriately low levels in the blood for the degree of anemia present;

(ii) reduced erythropoietic response of the bone marrow to ESA;

(iii) hepcidin-induced failure of iron absorption from the gut, and

(iv) hepcidin-induced trapping of iron in iron stores in the macrophages and hepatocytes.

Hepcidin [14, 15] is a protein released from the liver by IL-6. It inhibits the protein ferroportin, which is found in the gastrointestinal tract, macrophages and hepatocytes, and is responsible for the release of iron from these cells and tissues into the blood [see accompanying article by Nemeth and Ganz, pp 78–86]. Therefore, if ferroportin is inhibited, gastrointestinal iron absorption is diminished, and iron is also not released from its storage in macrophages and hepatocytes. Consequently, serum iron is decreased resulting in decreased delivery of iron to the bone marrow and therefore iron deficiency anemia, even in the presence of adequate total iron stores – the so-called functional iron deficiency. Since hepcidin is filtered and removed in the kidney, its levels increase in CKD, which can also partly explain the iron deficiency in CKD [16] and CHF. The inhibition of the bone marrow activity in

CHF caused by the cytokines may explain why CHF patients require very high doses of EPO to increase Hb, as their erythropoiesis is resistant to EPO therapy [17].

Interestingly, there may be a vicious circle operating, with cytokines causing low iron levels and low iron levels causing increased cytokine production [18]. Compared to hemodialysis patients taking EPO alone, those taking EPO and IV iron had lower proinflammatory TNF-α levels and higher anti-inflammatory cytokine IL-4 levels as well as lower levels of total peroxide (a marker of free radical concentration) [18].

Use of Angiotensin-Converting Enzyme Inhibitors (ACEI) and Angiotensin Receptor Blockers
These agents can cause reduced production of EPO and reduced activity of EPO in the bone marrow, since angiotensin is a stimulator of EPO production and erythropoiesis. ACEI can also increase the levels of erythropoietic inhibitors in the blood, further inhibiting erythropoiesis.

Hemodilution
It has been suggested that in many CHF cases anemia is partly due to hemodilution [19–21]. This has recently been further investigated by Abramov et al. [22]. It was found that a true red cell deficit was present in 88% of CHF patients with anemia and diastolic CHF and 59% of those with anemia and systolic CHF. All the systolic CHF patients and 71% of the diastolic CHF patients also had expanded plasma volume. This study suggests that there is a true red cell deficit in the majority of anemic CHF patients, but hemodilution is also very common.

Diabetes
The EPO-producing cells in the kidney may be damaged early by glycosylation, which can explain why, for the same degree of renal function, diabetics have a lower Hb than non-diabetics.

Gastrointestinal Problems
These include bleeding from aspirin, clopidogrel, warfarin-like agents, malignant tumors, polyps, esophagitis, or reduced iron absorption resulting from atrophic gastritis (which can also cause vitamin B_{12} deficiency), or from CHF-induced damage to the intestinal wall. It is also possible that proton pump inhibitors such as omeprazole, which are extremely widely used, reduce iron absorption [23].

Why Is Anemia Increasing in the CHF Population?

It is possible that the increase in the prevalence and severity of anemia which is being seen in CHF [11, 12] is due mainly to a combination of the increasing age of the population (age alone is associated with a lower Hb), the increasing prevalence of renal failure in CHF, the increasing prevalence of diabetes and the better care of CHF with ACEIs and angiotensin receptor blockers. All these could cause or worsen the anemia [4–12].

The Effect of Correction of Anemia in CHF Patients Treated with EPO

Studies of patients with CHF in whom the anemia has been treated have used either ESA, e.g. EPO, or its derivatives, the longer-acting darbepoetin (DA) or pegylated Mircera along with the addition of either oral or IV iron. Such treatment has been reported in uncontrolled studies [24–28], non-placebo-controlled studies [29–31], and small, single-blind [32–35] and double-blind [36, 37], placebo-controlled studies or larger, double-blind, placebo-controlled studies [38–40]. The Hb increased by an average of about 2 g/dl with ESA treatment. These studies resulted in the following findings.

Combined Mortality and CHF Hospitalization. Pooled analysis of 473 patients included in the Study of Anemia in Heart Failure-the Heart Failure Trial (STAMINA-HeFT) study, and another controlled trial of DA showed a strong trend to a reduced risk of the combined endpoint of all-cause mortality or first heart-failure-related hospitalization (hazard ratio 0.67; confidence interval 0.44–1.03; p = 0.06) in patients treated with ESA compared to placebo [41].

Reduced Hospitalization Alone. In a recent meta-analysis of seven of these randomized trials of ESA in CHF, including 363 treated patients and 287 controls, there was a significantly lower risk of CHF hospitalization with the treatment (relative risk 0.59; p = 0.006) [42].

Improved New York Heart Association (NYHA) Functional Class. The NYHA class decreased (improved) by an average of about one class with treatment (e.g. from 3 to 2) and remained unchanged in the control group. This represents a very significant degree of clinical improvement in the CHF symptoms of fatigue and shortness of breath with exertion and at rest.

Reduced β-Natriuretic Peptide Levels. They fell on average by about 250 pg/ml in ESA-treated patients in the studies in which it was assessed, a decrease of about 50%.

In the control group, it tended to increase (worsen). This test is an important measure of CHF severity as it measures pressure and volume overload and is one of the most accurate predictors of mortality and morbidity in CHF.

Increased Oxygen Consumption during Exercise. This increased on average by about 15% in the ESA group. This test is an important measure of CHF severity. In the control group, it was unchanged or worsened.

Increased Exercise Duration and Distance Walked. These two parameters of patient function increased on average by about 20% each in the treated group and remained unchanged in the control group.

Quality of Life. The average score was increased in the treated group according to the Kansas City Cardiomyopathy Questionnaire and the Patient Global Assessment Scale. It was unchanged in the control group.

Left-Ventricular Ejection Fraction. This increased on average by about 6% in the treatment group and was unchanged in the control group.

Comparison to Other Forms of CHF Therapy. The above functional changes produced by ESA are at least equal to those produced by ACEI [43] and β-blockers [44] in CHF, underlining the possible significance of correction of the anemia by ESA in CHF if these results are verified by larger studies.

Other Effects of EPO. In addition to the above findings, several of the studies have shown that correction of the anemia with ESA reduced diuretic dose, heart rate, plasma volume, left-ventricular hypertrophy and dilation, pulmonary artery pressure, the severity of mitral regurgitation, and inflammatory factors such as IL-6 and C-reactive protein, and improved renal function, caloric intake, depression, sleep apnea, left-ventricular diastolic function, and the adhesive and proliferative properties of circulating endothelial progenitor cells [24–37].

However, in three larger multicenter double-blind placebo-controlled studies using DA, no significant improvement was found in either the NYHA class, hospitalization or death [38–40], although some showed improved quality of life and improved renal function. In the largest study [40], in both the treatment and the control groups, the higher the increase in Hb, the greater was the improvement in exercise duration.

Adverse Effects. In a pooled analysis of all three DA studies including a total of 515 patients, there were no differences in the rate of adverse effects or death compared to placebo [45]. No differences occurred in mortality or in the incidence of hypertension, venous thrombosis, pulmonary embolus, cerebrovascular disorder, myocardial infarction, or other cardiovascular events.

The Effect of IV Iron Alone in the Anemia of CHF

Experimental studies in animals have shown that severe iron deficiency can cause diastolic dysfunction and heart failure with pulmonary congestion, left-ventricular hypertrophy and dilation, cardiac fibrosis, a reduction in EPO levels, a worsening of the molecular signaling pathways (as measured by cardiac STAT3 phosphorylation), an increase in the inflammatory cytokine TNF-α, and proteinuria [46]. In addition, iron deficiency in rat hearts causes mitochondrial ultrastructural aberrations, irregular sarcomere organization, and release of cytochrome C [47]. Beutler et al. [48] showed almost 50 years ago that iron deficiency can negatively affect enzymes throughout the body even without actual anemia being present. They also showed in a randomized double-blind placebo-controlled crossover study that oral iron can improve fatigue in non-anemic iron-deficient women [48, 49], and this has been subsequently confirmed by others [50, 51].

The prevalence of iron deficiency in CHF depends on how iron deficiency is defined. If merely defined as a percent transferrin saturation (%Tf_{Sat}) <16 it was found in one preliminary study in 78% of anemic and 61% of non-anemic patients, whereas if it was defined as a %Tf_{Sat} <16 and a serum ferritin of 30–100 μg/l it was found in only 15% of anemic and 20% of non-anemic CHF patients [52]. In another preliminary study, if iron deficiency was defined as ferritin <100 μg/l or ferritin 100–300 μg/l and %Tf_{Sat} ≤15% it was found in 61% of anemics and 43% of non-anemics [53]. In another study of anemia in CHF, about half the patients had serum iron below normal, and the great majority of anemic patients also had an elevated soluble transferrin receptor (a measure of iron deficiency) [54]. In a study of anemia in severe CHF, reduced iron stores in the bone marrow were found in 73% of the cases [55]. Therefore, pure iron deficiency (defined as a serum ferritin <100 μg/l and Tf_{Sat} <20%) or functional iron deficiency (defined as a serum ferritin >100 μg/l and %Tf_{Sat} <20%) are commonly seen in CHF patients with anemia or even without anemia. Does IV iron improve iron deficiency in these CHF patients?

Three recent studies on IV iron in anemic CHF patients, two uncontrolled studies [56, 57] and one double-blind placebo-controlled study [58], have shown improved Hb, left-ventricular ejection fraction, NYHA class, quality of life, left-ventricular hypertrophy and dilation, exercise capacity, renal function, as well as reduced heart rate, β-natriuretic peptide, C-reactive protein and hospitalization.

Silverberg/Wexler/Palazzuoli/Iaina/
Schwartz

In another recent CHF controlled study of IV iron in patients with iron deficiency with or without anemia, even though the Hb did not improve significantly with IV iron, there was still an improvement in NYHA class, patient global assessment, and oxygen consumption [59]. This suggests, as noted in the animal studies above, that part of the effect of iron on the heart may be related not only to the improved oxygenation from the increased Hb causing increased oxygen delivery to the cells, but also directly to the effects of iron on improving mitochondrial function, resulting in increased oxygen utilization, and ATP and energy production, unassociated with the correction of the anemia. A multicenter controlled study using IV iron alone in CHF is now in progress.

There is some evidence in hemodialysis patients that IV iron treatment is associated with a lower mortality [60–62]. Recently, in CKD patients not on dialysis, it was found that the lower the %Tf$_{Sat}$ the higher the mortality, again raising the possibility that iron deficiency may be a common and reversible cause of severe cardiovascular disease [63]. Although there has been concern about increased iron stores being associated with increased risk of coronary heart disease [64], this has not been confirmed by some recent studies [65] and the issue is still controversial.

In patients with CKD who are anemic but not in CHF, IV iron alone may also increase the Hb level significantly [66–69], discouraging the use of ESA altogether in many cases. Although there has been concern about IV iron causing renal disease [70], this has not been confirmed by most studies [58, 66, 68, 69]. However, IV iron can cause oxidative stress [71], and therefore long-term controlled studies of IV iron are needed to evaluate the effects of IV iron in CKD, as in CHF.

In most studies comparing oral to IV iron in CKD, IV iron has been found to produce a greater Hb response with fever side effects [68, 69]. Recently, new IV iron preparations have become available. To give 1,000 mg of elemental iron, ferric carboxymaltose and low-molecular-weight iron dextran can be given as a single injection, ferumoxytol would require 2 injections of about 500 mg each, and iron sucrose and ferric gluconate 5 injections of 200 mg each. If the safety of the new preparations which allow higher dosing is confirmed by further studies, this may render IV iron therapy more convenient.

Iron Deficiency and Thrombocytosis

The incidence of venous thromboembolism is greatly increased in CHF [72], and indeed CHF is considered to be a hypercoagulable state [73]. Could iron deficiency in these CHF patients be one cause of this? Iron deficiency can cause thrombocytosis which can lead to increased thrombosis, atherosclerosis, and increased mortality [74–76]. Correction of the iron deficiency with IV iron in EPO-treated dialysis patients reduced the platelet count significantly [77]. In a recent study (submitted for publication) in anemic CKD patients, we found that 22 patients who received 1,000-mg IV injections of iron without EPO in 5 weekly 200-mg doses had a significant fall in platelets of 10.5% by 1 week after the last injection. In another 55 patients who received this same iron dose but also 10,000 IU s.c. epoetin-β weekly for 5 weeks, Hb increased more than in the IV iron-EPO group but there was no significant change in the platelet count. The platelet count would have been expected to rise by 10% with EPO alone [78]. Thus IV iron prevented this rise in the EPO-treated group. This may be important, since thrombocytosis may be one of the missing links in causing the increased incidence of cardiovascular effects of EPO in cancer [75] and in CKD [74, 76]. High doses of EPO in CKD are associated with more iron deficiency, more severe thrombocytosis, and increased mortality [74]. Iron deficiency also increases oxidative stress [79].

A recent meta-analysis has shown that IV iron increases the Hb level to a greater extent than oral iron both in dialysis patients and in non-dialysis patients with CKD [69]. Addition of IV iron to hemodialysis patients resistant to EPO has increased Hb further and more rapidly, as well as the percentage of patients who reached the target Hb, facilitated a reduction in the EPO dose, and reduced adverse events compared to a control group even in patients whose %Tf$_{Sat}$ was initially up to 25% and serum ferritin initially 500–1,200 μg/l [80, 81].

Similarly, in the anemia of cancer patients who are on ESA, not only does IV iron raise the Hb level even higher and more rapidly, increase the percentage of patients who reach the target Hb, and reduce the EPO dose, but it also reduces total costs of care [82]. Since the high doses of EPO used in anemic cancer patients have been linked to increased spread of cancer, increased thrombophlebitic complications and increased mortality [82–84], there is growing interest in reducing the EPO doses by using more IV iron in these conditions. There is now a black box warning in cancer patients. FDA instructions require ESA to be withheld from patients whose Hb level exceeds 12 g/dl and high doses of ESA to be avoided.

Predicting Who Will Respond to IV Iron

There is no test that can predict with great accuracy the degree of response to IV iron in patients taking ESA in CKD [76, 85] or cancer [82]. Generally, in CKD the $\%Tf_{Sat}$ is a better predictor than ferritin, and the reticulocyte Hb is better than $\%Tf_{Sat}$ [76, 85, 86], but the differences are probably not large enough to be clinically useful.

The Non-Hematopoietic Biological Effects of EPO

The usefulness of ESA in CHF has been shown in animal studies where its use in CHF after myocardial infarction or after production of cardiac damage from other causes, with or without improving the Hb, has improved endothelial dysfunction, increased neovascularization of the heart muscle, and reduced apoptosis of cardiomyocytes, oxidative stress, inflammation, fibrosis, and hypoxic damage, and prevented functional impairment of the heart [87–89]. At least part of these effects is due to the increase in number and activity of endothelial progenitor cells from the bone marrow [87–89].

Other Potential Problems with EPO

High doses of ESA are potentially harmful for other reasons [90, 91]. These harmful effects include hypertension, which is probably directly due to ESA. The blood pressure response to EPO is related to the dose but not to the associated increase in Hb [90, 91]. ESA may cause hypertension by impairing NO production in the arteriole, by activating the renin-angiotensin-aldosterone system (RAAS) and the sympathetic system, and also by increasing endothelin, thromboxane, and prostaglandin $F_2\alpha$, and by lowering the release of prostacyclin. All of these can cause vasoconstriction and can increase the blood pressure.

ESA might also accelerate diabetic proliferative retinopathy and allograft renal artery stenosis [90].

ESA, as mentioned earlier, can also heighten inflammation via activation of cytokines and prothrombotic factors. It may cause thrombocytosis by enhancing the action of thrombopoietin and may also stimulate clot formation by stimulating the production of E selectin, P selectin, von Willebrand factor, and plasminogen activator inhibitor. All of these would cause an increase in clot formation [90] and, along with hypertension, promote atherosclerosis [90, 91]. At least part of the stimulation of the thrombocytosis and increased coagulation may be ascribed to – as mentioned earlier – the EPO-induced iron deficiency [90].

To What Level Should Hb Be Corrected?

US FDA guidelines for ESA products are available for CKD but not CHF. They state that dosing should be individualized to achieve and maintain Hb levels within the range of 10–12 g/dl and that high doses of these agents should be avoided [92]. The concern about higher Hb levels and about high doses of ESA in CKD patients has been triggered by the CHOIR (Correction of Hemoglobin and Outcomes in Renal Insufficiency) study, a study in ESA-treated patients both not on dialysis [93] and on hemodialysis [94], and by a meta-analysis of ESA in dialysis and non-dialysis renal failure [95], all of which have found increased adverse cardiovascular events in the higher Hb group. However, this has not been noted in any of the studies in CHF patients mentioned above that were treated with ESA and oral or IV iron and whose mean Hb values after treatment were between 12.5 and 14 g/dl. It may be that it is the high dose of ESA in renal failure patients resistant to lower doses that increases the cardiovascular risk rather than the high Hb level itself, since those who achieve the higher Hb levels without high doses of ESA actually have lower mortality and morbidity [74, 76, 93–96]. The relative contribution of high Hb levels and high ESA doses, however, is still unclear. Hopefully, the role of higher target Hb levels in CHF will be answered by the reduction in adverse events with DA-α in heart failure – the RED-HF (Reduction of Events with Darbepoetin-α in Heart Failure) study. The Data Monitoring Committee scrutinizing early results from this study, a double-blind multicenter placebo-controlled trial of DA in 3,400 anemic CHF patients, which now includes >1,000 patients treated for 6–18 months and has an Hb target of 13 g/dl, has found no evidence of increased frequency of adverse events in the treated group [pers. commun.].

A total of almost 4,000 patients have been entered in the current double-blind placebo-controlled TREAT (Trial to Reduce Cardiovascular Events with Aranesp Therapy) study of DA in non-dialyzed diabetic patients with renal insufficiency and an initial Hb of 9–11 g/dl [96]. The target Hb in the trial is 13 g/dl. The Data Safety Monitoring Board has thus far not recommended any change in the conduct of the study, suggesting that there is no excess of adverse events so far in the treated group.

How Does Anemia Worsen CHF?

This has been recently reviewed [5]. Anemia causes a fall in systemic vascular resistance due in part to the reduced viscosity of the blood and partly due to nitric oxide-mediated vasodilation caused by tissue hypoxia. The decrease in systemic vascular resistance reduces the blood pressure and causes activation of the baroreceptors. This baroreceptor activation activates the sympathetic system, the RAAS and vasopressin, and results in tachycardia and peripheral vasoconstriction; in addition, it leads to a decrease in renal blood flow and glomerular filtration rate. This causes salt and water retention and an increase in extracellular and plasma volume and β-natriuretic peptide – a sign of increased stretching of the cardiac muscle. All this can lead to left-ventricular dilation and hypertrophy and the production or worsening of CHF. Anemia has also been associated with elevated nocturnal blood pressure in hypertensive patients [97] and resistant hypertension [98] perhaps related to all the above factors.

The same activation of the sympathetic system, the RAAS system, and vasopressin are present in low-output CHF so that essentially two diseases are present, anemia and CHF, with similar pathophysiology, with both of them reducing renal function, and causing fluid retention and progressive cardiac damage. The fall in renal function in CHF may lead to progressive parenchymal damage as evidenced by progressively increasing proteinuria [99]. It is not surprising then that treatment of both CHF and anemia will be necessary to preserve cardiac and renal function.

The improvement in cardiac function seen with correction of the anemia may be due to many factors. Anemia causes tachycardia and tachycardia alone can have a profound negative effect on cardiac function in CHF [100, 101]. On the other hand, the reduction in heart rate with correction of the anemia may reduce myocardial oxygen consumption (the work of the heart) which can cause a great improvement in cardiac function [100, 101]. Correction of anemia in CHF with ESA or IV iron slows the heart rate [58, 102], which both reduces the work of the heart, and increases left-ventricular diastolic filling

and the time for diastolic coronary perfusion to take place. All of these improve myocardial ischemia. Another mechanism for the improvement in cardiac function is the improvement in Hb itself, which increases the oxygen supply to the heart. The improvement in anemia will reduce sympathetic, RAAS, and vasopressin activity and thus improve renal function, and prevent increased salt/water absorption, increased fluid load to the heart [5], and the toxic effects of these neurohormones on cardiac muscle. Finally, the direct cellular effects of ESA and IV iron on the myocardial cell may also improve cardiac function.

Experimental studies in animals suggest another factor contributing to myocardial damage in anemia. They show that the damaged heart goes into CHF at a higher Hb than the normal heart, suggesting that the damaged heart is more susceptible to anemia than the normal heart [103].

How Well Is the Anemia of CHF Being Investigated and Treated?

In a recent study of 11,754 US Medicare recipients in 2002 with both CKD and anemia but not on dialysis, 62% had CHF but only 7% of these CHF patients received ESA for it. Of the entire 11,754, only 38.4% had had an iron test performed during the year [104]. In a study of 6,159 CHF patients with stable heart failure at the Cleveland Clinic from 2001 to 2006 [105], 17.2% were found to be anemic initially, but documented evaluation of these patients was found in only 3% of cases, only 8% received ESA and only 21% received iron supplementation. In a study of 14,985 anemic CHF patients in various health care systems in the US in 2000, only 527 (3.5%) received ESA and only 22 (0.2%) received iron injections [106]. Thus it would appear that the anemia of CHF is grossly under-diagnosed, under-investigated, and under-treated.

Conclusions

Several but not all studies available to date seem to point to the importance of correcting anemia in patients with CHF with ESA and/or IV iron, but we must await the publication of larger, adequately powered placebo-controlled studies to be certain. What can at least be said for now is that the studies currently available in CHF seem to quite consistently show improvement in many crucial CHF parameters without adverse effects. Faced with patients who have both CHF and Hb <12 g/dl it may well be that ESA use should be considered to raise Hb to 12 g/dl. If iron deficiency is present, as it often is, correction of this with IV iron even without ESA may also be a useful intervention and might even become the first therapy applied. Correction of iron deficiency even without the presence of anemia may also be indicated, but here again data are lacking. Correction of iron deficiency also lowers the platelet count and prevents thrombocytosis seen in this condition. It may well turn out that a combined approach of ESA and IV iron is the best approach to correction of the anemia in CHF since this will allow a lower dose of both agents to be used. This will reduce the chances of side effects caused by high doses of either agent, reduce the dose and cost of ESA, cause a more rapid and greater Hb response than either agent alone, increase the chances of reaching the target hemoglobin, and reduce the chances of iron deficiency being induced by ESA which could cause resistance to ESA therapy, thrombocytosis, and its thromboembolic and atherosclerotic complications. Clearly, the relative role of ESA and IV iron in the treatment of the anemia of CHF merits further investigation.

References

1 Lloyd-Jones D, Adams R, Carnethon M, De Simone G, Ferguson TB, Flegal K, Ford E, Furie K, Go A, Greenlund K, Haase N, Hailpern S, Ho M, Howard V, Kissela B, Kittner S, Lackland D, Lisabeth L, Marelli A, McDermott M, Meigs J, Mozaffarian D, Nichol G, O'Donnell C, Roger V, Rosamond W, Sacco R, Sorlie P, Stafford R, Steinberger J, Thom T, Wasserthiel-Smoller S, Wong N, Wylie-Rosett J, Hong Y, American Heart Association Statistics Committee and Stroke Statistics Subcommittee: Heart disease and stroke statistics – 2009 update: a report from the American Heart Association Statistics Committee and Stroke Statistics Subcommittee. Circulation 2009;119:480–486.

2 Bleumink GS, Knetsch AM, Sturkenboom MC, Straus SM, Hofman A, Deckers JW, Witteman JC, Stricker BH: Quantifying the heart failure epidemic: prevalence, incidence rate, lifetime risk and prognosis of heart failure. The Rotterdam Study. Eur Heart J 2004; 25:1614–1619.

3 Beutler E, Waalen J: The definition of anemia: what is the lower limit of normal of the blood hemoglobin concentration. Blood 2006;107:1747–1750.

4 Silverberg DS, Wexler D, Iaina A, Schwartz D: The role of anaemia in patients with congestive heart failure: a short review. Eur J Heart Failure 2008;10:819–823.

5 Anand IS: Anemia and chronic heart failure. J Am Coll Cardiol 2008;52:501–511.

6 Mitchell JE: Emerging role of anemia in heart failure. Am J Cardiol 2007;99:15D–20D.

7 Silverberg DS, Wexler D, Iaina A, Schwartz D: The interaction between heart failure and other heart disease and anemia. Semin Nephrol 2006;26:296–306.

8 Tang YD, Katz SD: Anemia in chronic heart failure: prevalence, etiology, clinical correlates, and treatment options. Circulation 2006;113:2454–2461.

9 Kazory A, Ross EA: Anemia: the point of convergence or divergence for kidney disease and heart failure? J Am Coll Cardiol 2009;53:639–647.

10 Groenwald HF, Januzzi JL, Damman K, van Wijngaarden J, Hillege HL, van Veldhuisen DJ, van der Meer P: Anemia and mortality in heart failure patients: a systematic review and meta-analysis. J Am Coll Cardiol 2008; 52:818–827.

11 Owan TE, Hodge DO, Herges RM, Jacobsen SJ, Roger VL, Redfield MM: Secular trends in renal dysfunction in hospitalized heart failure patients. J Card Fail 2006;12:257–262.

12 Dunlay SD, Weston SA, Redfield MM, Killian JM, Roger VL: Anemia and heart failure: a community study. Am J Med 2008;121: 726–732.

13 Bansal N, Tighiouart H, Weiner D, Griffith J, Vlagopoulos P, Salem D, Levin A, Sarnak MJ: Anemia as a risk factor for kidney function decline in individuals with heart failure. Am J Cardiol 2007;99:1137–1142.

14 Nemeth E: Iron regulation and erythropoiesis. Curr Opin Hematol 2008;15:169–175.

15 Weiss G: Iron metabolism in the anemia of chronic disease. Biochim Biophys Acta 2009; 1790:682–693.

16 Ashby DR, Gale DP, Busbridge M, Murphy KG, Duncan ND, Cairns TD, Taube DH, Bloom SR, Tam FW, Chapman RS, Maxwell PH, Choi P: Plasma hepcidin levels are elevated but responsive to erythropoietin therapy in renal disease. Kidney Int 2009;75: 976–981.

17 Lopez-Gomez JM, Portoles JM, Aljama P: Factors that condition the response to erythropoietin in patients on hemodialysis and their relation to mortality. Kidney Int 2008; 74(suppl 11):S75–S81.

18 Weiss G, Meusburger E, Radacher G, Garimorth K, Neyer U, Mayer G: Effect of iron treatment on circulating cytokine levels in ESRD patients receiving recombinant human erythropoietin. Kidney Int 2003;64: 572–578.

19 Androne AS, Katz SD, Lund L, LaManca J, Hudaihed A, Hryniewicz K, Mancini DM: Hemodilution is common in patients with advanced heart failure. Circulation 2003; 107:226–229.

20 Westenbrink BD, Visser FW, Voors AA, Smilde TD, Lipsic E, Navis G, Hillege HL, van Gilst WH, van Veldhuisen DJ: Anaemia in chronic heart failure is not only related to impaired renal perfusion and blunted erythropoietin production, but to fluid retention as well. Eur Heart J 2007;28:166–171.

21 Adlbrecht C, Kommata S, Hulsmann M, Szekeres T, Bieglmayer C, Strunk G, Karanikas G, Berger R, Mörtl D, Kletter K, Maurer G, Lang IM, Pacher R: Chronic heart failure leads to an expanded plasma volume and pseudoanaemia, but does not lead to a reduction in the body's red cell volume. Eur Heart J 2008;29:2343–2350.

22 Abramov D, Cohen RS, Katz SD, Mancini D, Maurer MS: Comparison of blood volume characteristics in anemic patients with low versus preserved left ventricular ejection fraction. Am J Cardiol 2008;102:1069–1072.

23 Hutchinson C, Geissler CA, Powell JJ, Bomford A: Proton pump inhibitors suppress absorption of dietary non-haem iron in hereditary haemochromatosis. Gut 2007; 56: 1291–1295.

24 Silverberg DS, Wexler D, Blum M, Keren G, Sheps D, Leibovitch E, Brosh D, Laniado S, Schwartz D, Yachnin T, Shapira I, Gavish D, Baruch R, Koifman B, Kaplan C, Steinbruch S, Iaina A: The use of subcutaneous erythropoietin and intravenous iron for the treatment of the anemia of severe, resistant congestive heart failure improves cardiac and renal function and functional cardiac class, and markedly reduces hospitalizations. J Am Coll Cardiol 2000;35:1737–1744.

25 Silverberg DS, Wexler D, Blum M, Tchebiner JZ, Sheps D, Keren G, Schwartz D, Baruch R, Yachnin T, Shaked M, Schwartz I, Steinbruch S, Iaina A: The effect of correction of anaemia in diabetics and non-diabetics with severe resistant congestive heart failure and chronic renal failure by subcutaneous erythropoietin and intravenous iron. Nephrol Dial Transplant 2003;18:141–146.

26 Silverberg DS, Wexler D, Blum M, Iaina A, Sheps D, Keren G, Scherhag A, Schwartz D: Effects of treatment with epoetin beta on outcomes in patients with anaemia and chronic heart failure. Kidney Blood Press Res 2005;28:41–47.

27 Hampl H, Hennig L, Rosenberger C, Gogoli L, Riedel E, Scherhag A: Optimized heart failure therapy and complete anemia correction on left ventricular hypertrophy in nondiabetic and diabetic patients undergoing hemodialysis. Kidney Blood Press Res 2005; 28:353–362.

28 Hampl H, Hennig L, Rosenberger C, Amirkhalily M, Gogoll L, Riedel E, Scherhag A: Effects of optimized heart failure therapy and anemia correction with epoetin β on left ventricular mass in hemodialysis patients. Am J Nephrol 2005;25:211–220.

29 Silverberg DS, Wexler D, Sheps D, Blum M, Keren G, Baruch R, Schwartz D, Yachnin T, Steinbruch S, Shapira I, Laniado S, Iaina A: The effect of correction of mild anemia in severe, resistant congestive heart failure using subcutaneous erythropoietin and intravenous iron: a randomized controlled study. J Am Coll Cardiol 2001;37:1775–1780.

30 Pappas KD, Gouva CD, Katopodis KP, Nikolopoulos PM, Korantzopoulos PG, Michalis LK, Goudevenos JA, Siamopoulos KC: Correction of anemia with erythropoietin in chronic kidney disease (stage 3 and 4): effects on cardiac performance. Cardiovasc Drugs Ther 2008;22:37–44.

31 Cosyns B, Velez-Roa S, Droogmans S, Pierard LA, Lancellotti P: Effects of erythropoietin administration on mitral regurgitation and left ventricular remodeling in heart failure patients. Int J Cardiol, E-pub ahead of print.

32 Mancini DM, Katz SD, Lang CC, LaManca J, Hudaihed A, Androne AS: Effect of erythropoietin on exercise capacity in patients with moderate to severe chronic heart failure. Circulation 2003;107:294–299.

33 Kourea K, Parissis JT, Farmakis D, Panou F, Paraskevaidis I, Venetsanou K, Filippatos G, Kremastinos DT: Effects of darbepoetin-alfa on plasma pro-inflammatory cytokines, anti-inflammatory cytokine interleukin-10 and soluble Fas/Fas ligand system in anemic patients with chronic heart failure. Atherosclerosis 2008;199:215–221.

34 Parissis JT, Kourea K, Panou F, Farmakis D, Paraskevaidis I, Ikonomidis I, Filippatos G, Kremastinos DT: Effects of darbepoetin α on right and left ventricular systolic and diastolic function in anemic patients with

chronic heart failure secondary to ischemic or idiopathic dilated cardiomyopathy. Am Heart J 2008;155:751.e1–e7.

35 Kourea K, Parissis JT, Farmakis D, Paraskevaidis I, Panou F, Filippatos G, Kremastinos DT: Effects of darbepoetin-alpha on quality of life and emotional stress in anemic patients with chronic heart failure. Eur J Cardiovasc Prev Rehabil 2008;15:365–369.

36 Palazzuoli A, Silverberg D, Iovine F, Capobianco S, Giannotti G, Calabrò A, Campagna SM, Nuti R: Erythropoietin improves anemia, exercise tolerance, and renal function and reduces B-type natriuretic peptide and hospitalization in patients with heart failure and anemia. Am Heart J 2006;152:1096.e9–e15.

37 Palazzuoli A, Silverberg DS, Iovine F, Calabrò A, Campagna MS, Gallotta M, Nuti R: Effects of beta-erythropoietin treatment on left ventricular remodeling, systolic function and B-type natriuretic peptide levels in patients with the cardiorenal anemia syndrome. Am Heart J 2007;154:645.e9–e15.

38 Ponikowski P, Anker SD, Szachniewicz J, Okonko D, Ledwidge M, Zymlinski R, Ryan E, Wasserman SM, Baker N, Rosser D, Rosen SD, Poole-Wilson PA, Banasiak W, Coats AJ, McDonald K: Effect of darbepoetin alfa on exercise tolerance in anemic patients with symptomatic chronic heart failure: a randomized, double-blind, placebo-controlled trial. J Am Coll Cardiol 2007;49:753–762.

39 van Veldhuisen DJ, Dickstein K, Cohen-Solal A, Lok DJ, Wasserman SM, Baker N, Rosser D, Cleland JG, Ponikowski P: Randomized, double-blind placebo-controlled study to evaluate the effect of two dosing regimens of darbepoetin alfa in patients with heart failure and anaemia. Eur Heart J 2007;28: 2208–2216.

40 Ghali J, Anand I, Abraham WT, Fonarow GC, Greenberg B, Krum H, Massie BM, Wasserman SM, Trotman ML, Sun Y, Knusel B, Armstrong P, Study of Anemia in Heart Failure Trial (STAMINA-HeFT) Group: Randomized double-blind trial of darbepoetin alfa in patients with symptomatic heart failure and anemia. Circulation 2008;117:526–535.

41 Abraham WT, Klapholz M, Anand I, Knusel B, Rosser D, Baker N, Sun Y, Van Veldhuisen DJ: Safety and efficacy of darbepoetin alfa treatment in anemic patients with symptomatic heart failure: a pooled analysis of two randomized, double-blind, placebo-controlled trials. Eur Heart J 2007;27(suppl):166.

42 van der Meer P, Groenveld HF, Januzzi JL Jr, van Veldhuisen DJ: Erythropoietin treatment in patients with chronic heart failure: a meta-analysis. Heart 2009;95:1309–1314.

43 Abdulla J, Abildstrom SZ, Christensen E, Kober L, Torp-Pedersen C: A meta-analysis of the effect of angiotensin-converting enzyme inhibitors on functional capacity in patients with symptomatic left ventricular

systolic dysfunction. Eur J Heart Fail 2004;6: 927–935.

44 MacMahon S, Sharpe N, Doughty R: Randomized placebo-controlled trial of carvedilol in patients with congestive heart failure due to ischemic heart disease. Lancet 1997; 349:374–380.

45 Klapholz M, Abraham WT, Ghali JK, Ponikowski P, Knusel B, Wasserman SM, Sun Y, Van Veldhuisen DJ: Pooled safety analysis of darbepoetin alfa in the treatment of symptomatic heart failure (abstract). Eur Heart J 2008;29(suppl):507.

46 Naito Y, Tsujino T, Matsumoto M, Sakoda T, Ohyanagi M, Masuyama T: Adaptive response of the heart to long-term anemia induced by iron deficiency. Am J Physiol Heart Circ Physiol 2009;296:H585–H593.

47 Dong F, Zhang X, Culver B, Chew HG, Kelley RO, Ren J: Dietary iron deficiency induces ventricular dilation, mitochondrial ultrastructural aberrations and cytochrome C release: involvement of nitric oxide synthase and protein tyrosine nitration. Clin Sci (Lond)2005;109:277–286.

48 Beutler E, Larsh SE, Gurney CW: Iron therapy in chronically fatigued, nonanemic women: a double-blind study. Ann Intern Med 1960;52:378–394.

49 Beutler E: History of iron in medicine. Blood Cells Mol Dis 2002;29:297–308.

50 Brownlie T, Utermohlen V, Hinton PS, Giordano C, Haas JD: Marginal iron deficiency without anemia impairs aerobic adaptation among previously untrained women. Am J Clin Nutr 2002;75:733–742.

51 Verdon F, Burnand B, Stubi CL, Bonard C, Graff M, Michaud A, Bischoff T, de Vevey M, Studer JP, Herzig L, Chapuis C, Tissot J, Pécoud A, Favrat B: Iron supplementation for unexplained fatigue in non-anaemic women: double blind randomised placebo controlled trial. BMJ 2003;326:1124–1126.

52 Murphy CL, Fitzsimons EJ, Jardine AJ, Sattar N, Mcmurray JJV: Routine assessment of iron status in all patients with heart failure may identify those at risk of developing anemia. Eur J Heart Fail Suppl 2007;61:24.

53 Grzeslo A, Jankowska EA, Witkowski T, Majda J, Petruk-Kowalczyk J, Banasiak W, Ponikowski P: Iron deficiency is a common finding in patients with stable chronic heart failure. Eur J Heart Fail Suppl 2006;5:132.

54 Opasich C, Cazzola M, Scelsi L, De Feo S, Bosimini E, Lagioia R, Febo O, Ferrari R, Fucili A, Moratti R, Tramarin R, Tavazzi L: Blunted erythropoietin production and defective iron supply for erythropoiesis as major causes of anaemia in patients with chronic heart failure. Eur Heart J 2005;26: 2232–2237.

55 Nanas JN, Matsouka C, Karageorgopoulos D, Leonti A, Tsolakis E, Drakos SG, Tsagalou EP, Maroulidis GD, Alexopoulos GP, Kanakakis JE, Anastasiou-Nana MI: Etiology of anemia in patients with advanced heart failure. J Am Coll Cardiol 2006;48:2485–2489.

56 Bolger AP, Bartlett FR, Penston HS, O'Leary J, Pollock N, Kaprielian R, Chapman CM: Intravenous iron alone for the treatment of anemia in patients with chronic heart failure. J Am Coll Cardiol 2006;48:1225–1227.

57 Usmanov RI, Zueva EB, Silverberg DS, Shaked M: Intravenous iron without erythropoietin for the treatment of iron deficiency anemia in patients with moderate to severe congestive heart failure and chronic renal insufficiency. J Nephrol 2008;21:236–242.

58 Toblli J, Lombrana A, Duarte P, Di Gennaro F: Intravenous iron reduces NT-pro-brain natriuretic peptide in anemic patients with chronic heart failure and renal insufficiency. J Am Coll Cardiol 2007;50:1657–1665.

59 Okonko DO, Grzeslo A, Witkowski T, Mandal AK, Slater RM, Roughton M, Foldes G, Thum T, Majda J, Banasiak W, Missouris CG, Poole-Wilson PA, Anker SD, Ponikowski P: Effect of intravenous iron sucrose on exercise tolerance in anemic and nonanemic patients with symptomatic chronic heart failure and iron deficiency FERRIC-HF: a randomized, controlled, observer-blinded trial. J Am Coll Cardiol 2008;51:103–112.

60 Kalantar-Zadeh K, Regidor DL, McAllister CJ, Michael B, Warnock DG: Time-dependent associations between iron and mortality in hemodialysis patients. J Am Soc Nephrol 2005;16:3070–3080.

61 Feldman HI, Joffe M, Robinson B, Knauss J, Cizman B, Guo W, Franklin-Becker E, Faich G: Administration of parenteral iron and mortality among hemodialysis patients. J Am Soc Nephrol 2004;15:1623–1632.

62 Pollak VE, Lorch JA, Shukla R, Satwah S: The importance of iron in long-term survival of maintenance hemodialysis patients treated with epoetin-alfa and intravenous iron: analysis of 9.5 years of prospectively collected data. BMC Nephrol 2009;10:6.

63 Kovesdy CP, Estrada W, Ahmadzadeh S, Kalantar-Zadeh K: Association of markers of iron stores with outcomes in patients with nondialysis-dependent chronic kidney disease. Clin J Am Soc Nephrol 2009;4:435–441.

64 Tuomainen TP, Punnonen K, Nyyssonen K, Salonen JT: Association between body iron stores and the risk of acute myocardial infarction in men. Circulation 1998;97:1461–1466.

65 Sun Q, Ma J, Rifai N, Franco OH, Rexrode KM, Hu FB: Excessive body iron stores are not associated with risk of coronary heart disease in women. J Nutr 2008;138:2436–2441.

66 Mircescu G, Garneata L, Capusa C, Ursea N: Intravenous iron supplementation for the treatment of anemia in predialyzed chronic renal failure patients. Nephrol Dial Transplant 2006;21:120–124.

67 Gotloib L, Silverberg DS, Fudin R, Shostak A: Iron deficiency is a common cause of anemia in chronic kidney disease and can often be corrected with intravenous iron. J Nephrol 2006;19:161–167.

68 Van Wyck DB, Roppolo M, Martinez CO, Mazey RM, McMurray S, for the United States Iron Sucrose (Venofer) Clinical Trials Group: A randomized, controlled trial comparing IV iron sucrose to oral iron in anemic patients with nondialysis-dependent CKD. Kidney Int 2005;68:2846–2856.

69 Rozen-Zvi B, Gafter-Gvili A, Paul M, Leibovici L, Shpilberg O, Gafter U: Intravenous versus oral iron supplementation for the treatment of anemia in CKD: systematic review and meta-analysis Am J Kidney Dis 2008;52:897–906.

70 Bishu K, Agarwal R: Acute injury with intravenous iron and concerns regarding long-term safety. Clin J Am Soc Nephrol 2006;1(suppl 1):S19–S23.

71 Kuo KL, Hung SC, Wei YH, Tarng DC: Intravenous iron exacerbates oxidative DNA damage in peripheral blood lymphocytes in chronic hemodialysis patients. J Am Soc Nephrol 2008;19:1817–1826.

72 Darze ES, Latado AS, Guimarães AG, Guedes RA, Santos AB, de Moura SS, Passos LC: Incidence and clinical predictors of pulmonary embolism in severe heart failure patients admitted to a coronary care unit. Chest 2005;128:2576–2580.

73 Imberti D, Pierfranseschi MG, Falciani M, Prisco D: Venous thromboembolism prevention in patients with heart failure: an often neglected issue. Pathophysiol Haemost Thromb 2008;36:69–74.

74 Streja E, Kovesdy CP, Greenland S, Kopple JD, McAllister CJ, Nissenson AR, Kalantar-Zadeh K: Erythropoietin, iron depletion, and relative thrombocytosis: a possible explanation for hemoglobin-survival paradox in hemodialysis. Am J Kidney Dis 2008;52:727–736.

75 Littlewood TJ: Normalization of hemoglobin in patients with CKD may cause harm: but what is the mechanism? Am J Kidney Dis 2008;52:642–644.

76 Fishbane S: Erythropoiesis-stimulating agent treatment with full anemia correction: a new perspective. Kidney Int 2009;75:358–365.

77 Dahl NV, Henry DH, Coyne DW: Thrombosis with erythropoietic stimulating agents – does iron-deficient erythropoiesis play a role? Semin Dial 2008;21:210–211.

78 Eschbach JW, Abdulhadi MH, Browne JK, Delano BG, Downing MR, Egrie JC, Evans RW, Friedman EA, Graber SE, Haley NR, Korbet S, Krantz SB, Lundin AP, Nissenson AR, Ogden DA, Paganini EP, Rader B, Rutsky EA, Stivelman J, Stone WJ, Teschan P, Van Stone JC, Van Wyck DB, Zuckerman K, Adamson JW: Recombinant human erythropoietin in anemic patients with end-stage renal disease. Results of a phase III multicenter clinical trial. Ann Intern Med 1989;111:992–1000.

79 Nagababu E, Gulyani S, Earley CJ, Cutler RG, Mattson MP, Rifkind JM: Iron-deficiency anaemia enhances red blood cell oxidative stress. Free Radic Res 2008;42:824–829.

80 Coyne DW, Kapoian T, Suki W, Singh AK, Moran JE, Dahl NV, Rizkala AR, DRIVE Study Group: Ferric gluconate is highly efficacious in anemic hemodialysis patients with high serum ferritin and low transferrin saturation: results of the Dialysis Patients' Response to IV Iron with Elevated Ferritin (DRIVE) Study. J Am Soc Nephrol 2007;18:975–984.

81 Kapoian T, O'Mara NB, Singh AK, Moran J, Rizkala AR, Geronemus R, Kopelman RC, Dahl NV, Coyne DW: Ferric gluconate reduces epoetin requirements in hemodialysis patients with elevated ferritin. J Am Soc Nephrol 2008;19:372–379.

82 Katodritou E, Zervas K, Terpos E, Brugnara C: Use of erythropoiesis stimulating agents and intravenous iron for cancer and treatment-related anaemia: the need for predictors and indicators of effectiveness has not abated. Br J Hematol 2008;142:3–10.

83 Bennett CL, Silver SM, Djulbegovic B, Samaras AT, Blau CA, Gleason KJ, Barnato SE, Elverman KM, Courtney DM, McKoy JM, Edwards BJ, Tigue CC, Raisch DW, Yarnold PR, Dorr DA, Kuzel TM, Tallman MS, Trifilio SM, West DP, Lai SY, Henke M: Venous thromboembolism and mortality associated with recombinant erythropoietin and darbepoetin administration for the treatment of cancer-associated anemia. JAMA 2008;299:914–924.

84 Rizzo JD, Somerfield MR, Hagerty KL, Seidenfeld J, Bohlius J, Bennett CL, Cella DF, Djulbegovic B, Goode MJ, Jakubowski AA, Rarick MU, Regan DH, Lichtin AE: Use of epoetin and darbepoetin in patients with cancer: 2007 American Society of Hematology/American Society of Clinical Oncology clinical practice guideline update. Blood 2008;111:25–41.

85 Singh AK, Coyne DW, Shapiro W, Rizkala AR, DRIVE Study Group: Predictors of the response to treatment in anemic hemodialysis patients with elevated ferritin and low transferrin saturation. Kidney Int 2007;71:1163–1171.

86 Fishbane S, Galgano C, Langley RC, Canfield W, Maesaka JK: Reticulocyte hemoglobin content in the evaluation of iron status of hemodialysis patients. Kidney Int 1997;52:217–222.

87 Maiese K, Li F, Chong ZZ: New avenues of exploration for erythropoietin. JAMA 2005;293:90–95.

88 Arcasoy MO: The non-haematopoietic biological effects of erythropoietin. Br J Haematol 2008;141:14–31.

89 Rastogi S, Sharov VG, Mishra S, Sabbah HN: Darbepoetin-alpha prevents progressive left ventricular dysfunction and remodeling in nonanemic dogs with heart failure. Am J Physiol Heart Circ Physiol 2008;295:H2475–H2482.

90 Vaziri ND: Anemia and anemia correction: surrogate markers or causes of morbidity in chronic kidney disease. Nat Clin Pract Nephrol 2008;4:436–445.

91 Krapf R, Hulter HN: Arterial hypertension induced by erythropoietin and erythropoiesis-stimulating agents (ESA). Clin J Am Soc Nephrol 2009;4:470–480.

92 US Food and Drug Administration: Information for Healthcare Professionals. Erythropoiesis Stimulating Agents (ESA). FDA Alert, 2007. http://www.fda.gov/cder/drug/InfoSheets/HCP/RHE200711HCP.htm

93 Singh AK, Szczech L, Tang KL, Barnhart H, Sapp S, Wolfson M, Reddan D, CHOIR Investigators: Correction of anemia with epoetin alfa in chronic kidney disease. N Engl J Med 2006;355:2085–2098.

94 Besarab A, Bolton WK, Browne JK, Egrie JC, Nissenson AR, Okamoto DM, Schwab SJ, Goodkin DA: The effects of normal as compared with low hematocrit values in patients with cardiac disease who are receiving hemodialysis and epoetin. N Engl J Med 1998;339:584–590.

95 Phommintikul A, Haas HJ, Elsik M, Krum H: Mortality and target haemoglobin concentrations in anaemic patients with chronic kidney disease treated with erythropoietin: a meta-analysis. Lancet 2007;369:381–388.

96 Pfeffer MA: Anemia treatment in chronic kidney disease: shifting uncertainty. Heart Failure Review 2008;13:425–430.

97 Marketou M, Patrianakos A, Parthenakis F, Zacharis E, Arfanakis D, Kochiadakis G, Chlouverakis G, Vardas P: Systemic blood pressure profile in hypertensive patients with low hemoglobin concentrations. Int J Cardiol, E-pub ahead of print.

98 Paul B, Wilfred NC, Woodman R, Depasquale C: Prevalence and correlates of anaemia in essential hypertension. Clin Exp Pharmacol Physiol 2008;35:1461–1464.

99 Smilde TDJ, Damman K, van der Harst P, Navis G, Daan Westenbrink B, Voors AA, Boomsma F, van Veldhuisen DJ, Hillege HL: Differential associations between renal function and 'modifiable' risk factors in patients with chronic heart failure. Clin Res Cardiol 2009;98:121–129.

100 Logeart D, Gueffet JP, Rouzet F, Pousset F, Chavelas C, Solal AC, Jondeau G: Heart rate per se impacts cardiac function in patients with systolic heart failure and pacing: a pilot study. Eur J Heart Fail 2009;11:53–57.

101 Fox K, Borer JS, Camm AJ, Danchin N, Ferrari R, Lopez Sendon JL, Steg PG, Tardif JC, Tavazzi L, Tendera M, Heart Rate Working Group: Resting heart rate in cardiovascular disease. J Am Coll Cardiol 2007;50:823–830.

102 Vaisman N, Silverberg DS, Wexler D, Niv E, Blum M, Keren G, Soroka N, Iaina A: Correction of anemia in patients with congestive heart failure increases resting energy expenditure. Clin Nutr 2004;23:355–361.

103 Levy PS, Kim SJ, Eckel PK, Chavez R, Ismail EF, Gould SA, Ramez Salem M, Crystal GJ: Limit to cardiac compensation during acute isovolemic hemodilution: influence of coronary stenosis. Am J Physiol 1993;265:H340–H349.

104 Collins AJ, Guo H, Gilbertson DT, Bradbury BD: Predictors of ESA use in the non-dialysis chronic kidney disease population with anemia. Nephron Clin Pract 2009;111:c141–c148.

105 Tang WH, Tong W, Jain A, Francis GS, Harris CM, Young JB: Evaluation and long-term prognosis of new-onset, transient, and persistent anemia in ambulatory patients with chronic renal failure. J Am Coll Cardiol 2008;51:569–576.

106 Nissenson AR, Wade S, Goodnough T, Knight K, Dubois RW: Economic burden of anemia in an insured population. J Manag Care Pharm 2005;11:565–574.

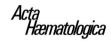

Acta Haematol 2009;122:120–133
DOI: 10.1159/000243796

Published online: November 10, 2009

Mitochondrial Iron Metabolism and Sideroblastic Anemia

Alex D. Sheftel[a]   Des R. Richardson[b]   Josef Prchal[c]   Prem Ponka[d]

[a]Institut für Zytobiologie, Philipps-Universität-Marburg, Marburg, Deutschland; [b]Department of Pathology and Bosch Institute, University of Sydney, Sydney, N.S.W., Australia; [c]Hematology Division, University of Utah, Salt Lake City, Utah, USA; and [d]Departments of Physiology and Medicine, McGill University and Lady Davis Institute for Medical Research, Jewish General Hospital, Montreal, Que., Canada

Key Words

ALAS2 · ABCB7 · Mitochondrial iron metabolism · Ring sideroblasts · Sideroblastic anemias · Transferrin

Abstract

Sideroblastic anemias are a heterogeneous group of disorders, characterized by mitochondrial iron overload in developing red blood cells. The unifying characteristic of all sideroblastic anemias is the ring sideroblast, which is a pathological erythroid precursor containing excessive deposits of non-heme iron in mitochondria with perinuclear distribution creating a ring appearance. Sideroblastic anemias may be hereditary or acquired. Hereditary sideroblastic anemias are caused by defects in genes present on the X chromosome (mutations in the ALAS2, ABCB7, or GRLX5 gene), genes on autosomal chromosomes, or mitochondrial genes. Acquired sideroblastic anemias are either primary (refractory anemia with ring sideroblasts, RARS, representing one subtype of the myelodysplastic syndrome) or secondary due to some drugs, toxins, copper deficiency, or chronic neoplastic disease. The pathogenesis of mitochondrial iron loading in developing erythroblasts is diverse. Ring sideroblasts can develop as a result of a heme synthesis defect in erythroblasts (ALAS2 mutations), a defect in iron-sulfur cluster assembly, iron-sulfur protein precursor release from mitochondria (ABCB7 mutations), or by a defect in intracellular iron metabolism in erythroid cells (e.g. RARS).

Copyright © 2009 S. Karger AG, Basel

Introduction

Sideroblastic anemias are a diverse group of disorders with several features in common. First of all, these anemias share an illuminating sign of ringed sideroblasts in the bone marrow. Additional common characteristics of sideroblastic anemias consist of hypochromic erythrocytes (however, some types are accompanied by macrocytic, in addition to microcytic, erythrocytes), increased plasma iron levels and transferrin (Tf) saturation, and erythroid hyperplasia of the bone marrow. The hallmark of the sideroblastic anemia, the ring sideroblast, is a pathological erythroid precursor containing excessive deposits of non-heme iron in mitochondria that can be visualized using transmission electron microscopy. However, Prussian blue staining can also reveal iron-overloaded mitochondria in ring sideroblasts. Iron-laden mitochondria display perinuclear distribution accounting for the ring appearance of sideroblasts. As will be dis-

Prof. Prem Ponka, MD, PhD
Lady Davis Institute for Medical Research
3755 Côte Ste-Catherine
Montreal, QC H3T 1E2 (Canada)
Tel. +1 415 340 8260, Fax +1 415 340 7502, E-Mail prem.ponka@mcgill.ca

cussed later, it seems that the pathogenesis of mitochondrial iron loading is not identical in all types of sideroblastic anemias. It is of considerable interest to mention that iron accumulation within mitochondria is an unusual pathological phenomenon occurring only in erythroblasts of patients with sideroblastic anemias and, to a much lesser degree, in cardiomyocytes of patients with Friedreich ataxia [1]. Mitochondrial iron accumulation has not been demonstrated in patients with either primary or secondary iron overload. It needs to also be pointed out that these pathological ring sideroblasts differ from sideroblasts which are present in normal bone marrow where normally 20–80% of the nucleated red cells possess iron-containing granules. Iron in these normal sideroblasts is in the form of cytosolic ferritin and can also be stained with Prussian blue. The number of these sideroblasts is directly proportional to the percentage of Tf saturated with iron.

Sideroblastic anemias may be acquired or hereditary. Acquired sideroblastic anemias are either primary (in which case these are clonal diseases [2], representing one subtype of the myelodysplastic syndromes, refractory anemia with ring sideroblasts, RARS) or secondary due to some drugs, toxins, copper deficiency, or chronic neoplastic disease [3] (table 1). Hereditary sideroblastic anemias are caused by defects in genes present on the X chromosome, autosomal chromosomes, or by defects in mitochondrial genes [3] (table 1).

Recently, several outstanding reviews dealing with sideroblastic anemias have been published [6–8].

Iron Transport, Storage, and Homeostatic Regulation

In order to understand the metabolic processes involved in the pathogenesis of sideroblastic anemias and other disorders leading to mitochondrial iron overload, an understanding of cellular iron metabolism is essential.

Iron is transported in the blood bound to the glycoprotein, Tf, which binds two ferric ions (fig. 1) [9]. Entry of iron into the cell occurs when two molecules of diferric-Tf form a complex with the Tf receptor 1 (TfR1) on the cell surface. The Tf-TfR1 complex is then internalized within an endosome and iron is released from Tf by a decrease in intravesicular pH mediated by a proton pump (fig. 1) [9, 10]. Iron is then reduced to its ferrous form probably by a ferric reductase enzyme known as Steap3 [11]. Fe^{2+} is then transported across the endosomal membrane by the divalent metal transporter-1 (DMT1; fig. 1) [12]. Once within the cytosol, iron is available for cellular processes and becomes part of a very poorly characterized compartment known as the chelatable iron pool or labile iron pool (LIP) [13].

The nature of the LIP remains controversial, but was originally thought to be composed of low-molecular-weight complexes of iron bound to citrate, amino acids, and ATP for example. However, more recently, the existence of a LIP that exists as a quantitatively significant intracellular pool of low M_r complexes has not been verified in erythroid cells where low M_r cellular iron behaved as an end-product rather than an intermediate [14]. Considering this, a model of iron trafficking requiring direct protein-protein interactions was proposed that could involve interactions of organelles [14, 15]. Other studies by several authors have provided evidence in erythroid cells that Tf-containing endosomes may transfer iron directly to the mitochondrion ('kiss and run' hypothesis), or to a site in close proximity to the latter organelle [16]. Evidence for alteration in the trafficking of iron is found in models of Friedreich's ataxia [17]. The absence of frataxin expression results in iron being vectored towards the mi-

Table 1. Classification of sideroblastic anemias

I *Acquired*
  A RARS
    (1) Subunit 1 of the mitochondrial cytochrome oxidase (?)
  B Sideroblastic anemia secondary to
    (1) Isoniazid
    (2) Pyrazinamide
    (3) Cycloserine
    (4) Chloramphenicol
    (5) Ethanol
    (6) Lead
    (7) Chronic neoplastic disease
    (8) Copper deficiency
    (9) D-Penicillamine

II *Hereditary*
  A X chromosome-linked
    (1) ALAS2 deficiency
    (2) Hereditary sideroblastic anemia with ataxia: mitochondrial ATP binding cassette (*ABCB7*) mutations
  B Autosomal
    (1) MLASA (*PUS1* mutations)
    (2) GLRX5 deficiency [4]
    (3) SLC25A38 mutations [5]
  C Mitochondrial
    (1) Pearson marrow-pancreas syndrome

Adapted from Beutler [3].

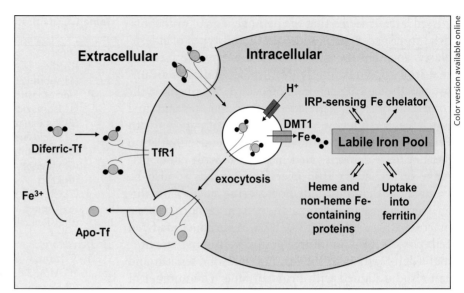

Fig. 1. Diagram illustrating Fe uptake from Tf by mammalian cells [63].

tochondrion and away from the cytosol that leads to mitochondrial iron overload [17, 67].

Irrespective of the mechanism of iron trafficking within the intracellular pool, it is used for incorporation into heme or iron-sulfur clusters (Fe/S; see Mitochondrial Iron Metabolism) or becomes stored in the multimeric iron storage protein, ferritin. Iron can also be released from cells by the plasma membrane protein, ferroportin, which transports iron from the inside to the outside of the cell [18]. How ferroportin transports iron to the cell surface remains unclear, although it is probably transported by this protein in the ferrous state.

The LIP has been thought to provide a rapidly adjustable source of iron for immediate metabolic utilization and is thought to be sensed by iron-regulatory proteins (IRPs). These are well-characterized mRNA-binding molecules that control the expression of molecules involved in iron uptake, utilization, and storage. Systemic regulation of iron absorption and cellular uptake is possible through both transcriptional and post-transcriptional mechanisms [18, 19]. IRP1 and IRP2 are important components of post-transcriptional regulation. The IRPs bind to iron-responsive elements (IREs), which are motifs present in the 3'- or 5'-untranslated region (UTR) of mRNA encoding proteins involved in the metabolism of iron. IRP1 is only active as an mRNA-binding protein when intracellular iron levels are low, as it otherwise contains a [4Fe-4S] cluster that prevents its binding to IREs. Similarly, IRP2 levels are severely decreased in iron-repleted cells as it is degraded under this condition by the proteasome. Of interest, it has been proposed that IRP2

is the major active RNA-binding protein in vivo, with IRP1 playing a lesser, but still significant role [20].

As an example of this type of regulation, under conditions of iron deprivation, IRP1 and IRP2 bind to the 3'-UTR of *DMT1* and *TfR1* mRNA and to the 5'-UTR of *ferritin, ferroportin (Fpn1)* mRNA, and erythroid-specific *ALAS* mRNA *(ALAS2)* [21]. Binding of IRPs to the 3' IRE stabilizes the mRNA and prevents it from being degraded, while binding to the 5' IRE blocks translation of the mRNA. Consequently, in response to iron deficiency, there is increased expression of DMT1 and TfR1 and the concomitant reduction in Fpn1, ferritin, and ALAS2 protein levels; this reduces iron export and storage to maximize the intracellular availability of iron for the increased metabolic needs of the cell. In contrast, enlargement of the LIP inactivates IRP1 binding to the IREs and promotes proteosomal catabolism of IRP2, resulting in augmented translation of ferritin and rapid degradation of transferrin receptor mRNA. This post-transcriptional system of reciprocal regulation of the proteins of uptake and storage/release enables a tight homeostatic control of intracellular iron metabolism.

Although it is generally assumed that the above-discussed IRE/IRP mechanism coordinates regulation of iron uptake and storage by all cells, there are some features of erythroid TfR regulation suggesting a distinct regulation of this receptor in these cells. Whereas in nonerythroid cells the transcriptional control of TfR expression in response to altered growth rates or iron deprivation does not seem to play a significant role, TfR is transcriptionally regulated and 'overexpressed' in chick embryo erythroblasts as well as MEL cells induced to synthesize hemoglobin [for review, see ref. 15]. This unique regulation is likely due to the fact that the TfR1 gene promoter contains an erythroid active element [22], which stimulates receptor gene transcription upon induction of hemoglobin synthesis. Since sideroblastic anemia is a result of disturbed iron metabolism in red cells, it is crucial to consider the erythroid-specific regulation of TfR1, the gateway for iron entry into these cells.

It is notable that the IRP-IRE system is not the only mechanism of regulating intracellular iron levels, with the low M_r peptide hormone, hepcidin, playing an essential role at the systemic level [23]. The regulation of hepcidin metabolism is reviewed by Elizabeta Nemeth and Tomas Ganz in an accompanying article in this issue [pp 78–86]. It is noteworthy that recent studies have revealed that like many other hormones, hepcidin is bound to a specific carrier protein, namely α_2-macroglobulin [24].

While dietary iron uptake is a crucial process, the recycling of hemoglobin iron from senescent red blood cells yields far greater amounts of the metal [25]. In fact, up to 30 times more iron is made available through the phagocytosis of aged erythrocytes by macrophages than is absorbed through the diet. This observation is in line with the fact that iron bound to hemoglobin in erythrocytes accounts for approximately two-thirds of total body iron.

Mitochondrial Iron Metabolism

Although some metalloenzymes directly incorporate iron into their protein backbone, the vast majority of iron-containing proteins wield the metal within the prosthetic groups of heme and/or iron-sulfur clusters (Fe/S). Mitochondria are the exclusive sites of heme synthesis as well as the major (if not exclusive) producers of Fe/S. Thus, the majority of functional iron within a cell is processed, if not resident, within these organelles. Because mitochondria are privy to the cytoavailability of iron, they are in an opportune setting to exert regulation upon iron homeostasis for the entire cell. The following section will discuss the iron anabolic pathways within mitochondria, how the mitochondria handle iron, and how mitochondria influence cellular iron metabolism.

Heme Biosynthesis
The production of heme (Fe[II]-protoporphyrin IX, PPIX) begins with a series of seven enzyme-catalyzed reactions to generate PPIX, which is then charged with Fe^{2+}

by ferrochelatase (FC). The first step in PPIX production, the condensation of glycine and succinyl coenzyme A to form 5-aminolevulinic acid (ALA), is catalyzed by ALA synthase (ALAS), which resides within the mitochondrial matrix. Mammals possess two isoforms of ALAS, a ubiquitous version that is required for 'housekeeping' heme synthesis in all tissues (ALAS1; encoded on chromosome 3) and an erythroid-specific version (ALAS2; encoded on the X chromosome) that is responsible for the enormously high demands for heme during erythropoiesis. The relevance of this important difference between erythroid and non-erythroid cells is discussed below (Etiology and Pathogenesis of Ring Sideroblast Formation). Once formed, ALA is somehow delivered to the cytosol, where four enzyme-catalyzed reactions produce coproporphyrinogen III, which is then somehow delivered to the mitochondria. In the mitochondria, coproporphyrinogen III is converted to protoporphyrinogen IX and then to PPIX. The final step in the production of heme is catalyzed by FC, which is associated with the inner mitochondrial membrane, its active site in the mitochondrial matrix (fig. 2).

Deficiencies in any of the eight enzymes of the heme biosynthetic pathway other than ALAS result in porphyrias (reviewed in Ajioka and Kushner [26]), owing to the direct toxicity of free porphyrins. Accordingly, it is expected that the levels of each enzyme downstream of ALA production are sufficient to prevent accumulation of intermediates. FC is no exception to this and will continue to convert PPIX to metalloporphyrin even when iron is not obtainable, using zinc(II) as a substitute for Fe^{2+}. Thus, erythrocyte zinc protoporphyrin (ZnPP) levels are generally indicative of the availability of Fe for FC. Such is the case in iron deficiency anemia. Care must be taken when considering reports referring to 'free erythrocyte protoporphyrin' or 'FEP', as, in many studies, this value is in fact ZnPP, and not bona fide free PPIX, which is generally found only under conditions of compromised FC activity. Such is generally the case in erythropoietic protoporphyria (EPP). Classical, hereditary EPP is autosomal dominant, but patients exhibit 75–90% reductions in FC activity.

Fe/S Protein Biogenesis (fig. 3)
In vitro, in the absence of oxygen, Fe/S will form spontaneously from sulfane sulfur (S^{2-}) and Fe^{2+}. However, under the conditions within living cells, reduced iron and sulfur are both unstable and potentially toxic. Hence, specialized biosynthetic systems have evolved to generate these metallocofactors. Most of our current knowledge of

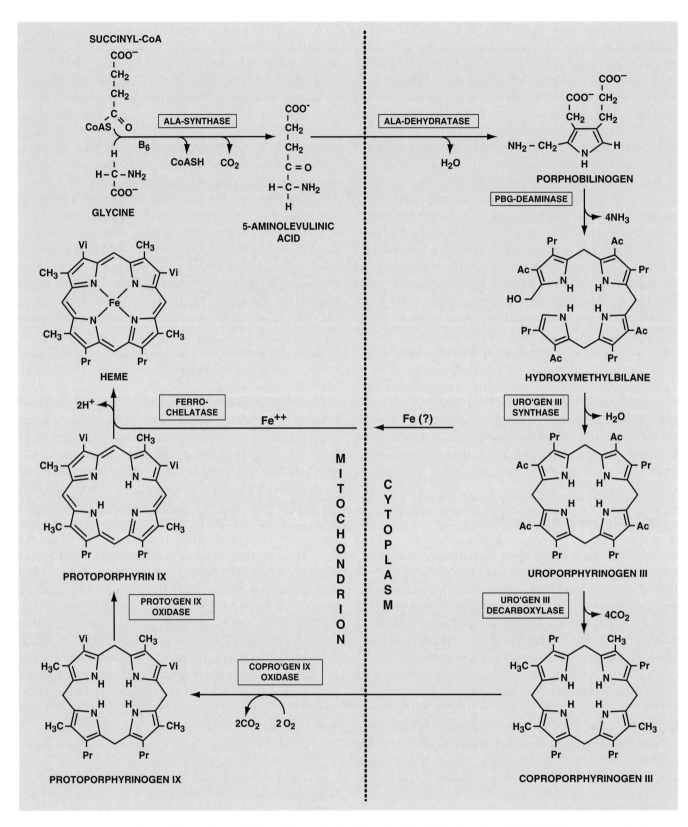

Fig. 2. The pathway of heme biosynthesis. B6 = Pyridoxal-5'-phosphate; URO'GEN = uroporphyrinogen; COPRO'GEN = coproporphyrinogen; PROTO'GEN = protoporphyrinogen; Ac = acetate; Pr = propionate; Vi = vinyl.

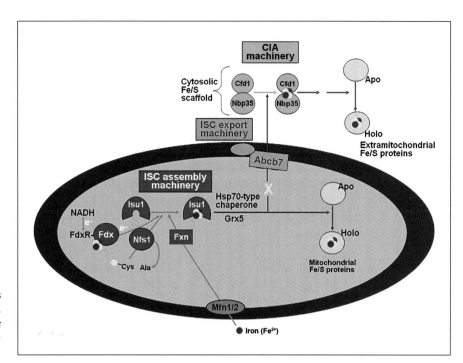

Fig. 3. Simplified Fe/S protein biogenesis schematic (please refer to main text). Fxn = Frataxin; X = unknown substrate exported by Abcb7. Cfd1/Nbp35 are a cytosolic scaffold complex [27].

Fe/S protein production stems from research in bacteria and yeast; however, current research efforts are providing increasing numbers of reports documenting functional conservation in mammals of the proteins involved. The subject of Fe/S protein biogenesis is the dedicated topic of some recent reviews [27] and is briefly discussed below.

The formation of a transient Fe/S on the scaffold protein, Isu1, requires the two elemental components to be in their reduced oxidation states. Sulfur is initially derived from cysteine via the cysteine desulfurase, Nfs1 [27, 28], to form alanine and persulfidic sulfur. This sulfur is then reduced, presumably by the ferredoxin (Fdx1 or Fdx1L)-Fdx reductase system that extracts electrons from NADH [27], and combined with iron on Isu1. Importantly, Fdx1 harbors a [2Fe-2S] of its own. The delivery of iron to Isu1 is not well understood, but is thought to involve frataxin, possibly as the iron donor [27]. Regardless, frataxin plays a critical role in the early stages of Fe/S protein biogenesis [29]. Isu1 serves only as a cluster for de novo cluster production from which an Hsp70-type chaperone system transfers the new clusters to apoproteins [27]. The monothiol glutaredoxin, Grx5, is also thought to participate in the delivery of clusters from Isu1 [27, 30].

Fe/S proteins also have important roles outside of the mitochondria. Several cytosolic proteins have recently been shown to play specialized roles in the formation of cytosolic and nuclear Fe/S proteins [27]. The mitochondria are indispensable for the de novo formation of all cellular Fe/S proteins since, if for no other reason, the only functional Nfs1 resides within these organelles [28]. In addition, in yeast cells, it appears that all of the aforementioned mitochondrial components are required for the formation of extramitochondrial Fe/S proteins [27, 31]. Frataxin, in mammals [29], and Grx5, in zebrafish [30], have also been shown to be required for extramitochondrial Fe/S proteins. There are two likely explanations for these findings: (1) Fe/S are generated inside mitochondria and then transported to the cytosol; (2) the formation and/or transport of an Fe/S precursor that is exported to the cytosol requires an intramitochondrial Fe/S protein. Since Fdx is required for Fe/S formation on Isu1 and contains a cluster, further characterization of the precise molecular function of Fdx in Fe/S protein biogenesis and/or identification of the exported moiety from mitochondria are required before it will be possible to rule out either of these hypotheses.

Mitochondrial Ferritin

In 2001, Levi et al. [32] reported the discovery of a mitochondrial version of the iron sequestration protein ferritin. Termed 'mitochondrial ferritin' (MFt), this protein is encoded by an intronless gene located on chromosome 5. MFt most closely resembles the cytosolic ferritin heavy chain, has ferroxidase activity, and forms a polymer capable of storing iron. Normally, the protein is only abundant in testes [32] and somewhat present in tissues of high metabolic activity, but it has also been observed to be elevated and storing iron in ring sideroblasts of patients with ALAS2 defects and RARS [33]. It has not yet been investigated whether MFt accumulates in ring sideroblasts of patients with X-linked sideroblastic anemia with ataxia (XLSA/A), or patients with Pearson marrow-pancreas syndrome, or those with mitochondrial myopathy and sideroblastic anemia (MLASA). Neither the function of MFt nor its regulation are yet understood.

Mitochondrial Transport of Iron

The only known mitochondrial iron import proteins identified so far in mammalian cells are the mitoferrins (Mfn). Mutation in the erythroid-specific Mfn isoform (Mfn1) caused microcytic, hypochromic anemia in a zebrafish model (frascati) [34]. In contrast to Mfn1, Mfn2, encoded by a separate gene, appears to be a ubiquitously expressed protein responsible for mitochondrial iron uptake in non-erythroid tissues [34]. Importantly, regulation of Mfn has not yet been reported under any conditions.

Interestingly, a group of patients with a variant of EPP has been discovered to harbor mutations in Mfn1 [35]. Presumably, the entry of iron is diminished in the developing red cells in these individuals, resulting in a two-pronged interference with the formation of heme from PPIX: (1) mitochondrial iron as a substrate for FC is reduced, and (2) iron is unavailable for the formation of Fe/S on FC. Human FC is an Fe/S protein containing a single, C-terminal [2Fe-2S] cluster which is required for the activity of the enzyme [36]. Another variant of EPP has recently been reported in a population of South African patients who are afflicted by a gain-of-function mutation in ALAS2 [37]. These patients have considerably elevated erythrocyte ZnPP as well as free PPIX levels but lack the iron loading seen in XLSA patients with mutations in ALAS2. It is important to note that while FC mutations were ruled out as contributing to the EPP of patients with Mfn1 mutations, it remains to be determined whether gain-of-function ALAS2 mutations may be present.

As mentioned above, a hitherto enigmatic compound is exported from mitochondria for the generation of cytosolic and nuclear Fe/S proteins. Three peptidic components facilitating this export function have been identified: the ATP-binding cassette protein ABCB7, a soluble, inner membrane space sulfhydryl oxidase Erv1, and glutathione [27]. ABCB7 is the central component in this export machinery. When its levels are reduced in cultured cells by RNA interference, iron accumulates in mitochondria [38]. Interestingly, ABCB7 deficiency in humans (three families have been discovered so far) results in XLSA/A [39, 40]. Although ring sideroblasts are present in these patients and mitochondrial iron deposition is present in mice with targeted deletion of ABCB7 in erythroid tissues [41], mice with liver-specific ablation of ABCB7 exhibit iron deposits that appear to be outside of mitochondria [40].

The mechanism of iron accumulation in mitochondria of ABCB7 deficiency has not been elucidated. In yeast, depletion of nearly all of the mitochondrial components of Fe/S protein biogenesis results in massive loading of mitochondria with iron [31]; however, the molecular mechanism responsible for this phenomenon also has yet to be understood. What is clear in both yeast and mammalian cells is that mitochondrial Fe/S protein biogenesis is required for appropriate regulation of cellular iron uptake. In vertebrates, IRP1 is erroneously activated under conditions of compromised mitochondrial or cytosolic Fe/S protein production [28, 30, 31], since the absence of [4Fe-4S] on the protein renders it able to bind IREs. There is also a link between heme synthesis and mitochondrial iron accumulation, at least in erythroid tissues, as chemical inhibitors of PPIX synthesis (isonicotinic acid hydrazide and succinylacetone) [14, for review see ref. 15], ALAS2 deficiency (sideroblastic anemia), and FC deficiency (classical EPP) [42] all can result in mitochondrial iron accumulation in developing red blood cells. In a recent paper, Guernsey et al. [5] described another SLC25 family transporter, which is mutated in patients with congenital sideroblastic anemia, that is required for heme biosynthesis. When the homologous transporter was ablated from yeast, ALA levels were diminished, suggesting that this transporter is required for ALA synthesis. They conjectured that this protein may be translocating glycine into mitochondria. Altogether, the inability to form Fe/S proteins and/or heme results in an iron-starved phenotype in mitochondria, resulting in acquisition and/or retention of the metal within the organelles. Deletion of a yeast homolog of another member of the SLC25 family of proteins, SLC25A39, has been shown to result in mitochondrial iron accumulation which caused iron to be incorporated into superoxide dismutase isoform 2 (SOD2) instead of manganese [43]. Further study in yeast revealed that there are at least two pools of iron within iron-overloaded mitochondria, one

Fig. 4. A model for the terminal mitochondrial-associated steps in the heme biosynthesis pathway. The post-endosomal path of iron in the developing red blood cells remains elusive or is, at best, controversial. Recent research supports the hypothesis that in erythroid cells a transient mitochondrion-endosome interaction is involved in iron translocation to its final destination. It has been proposed that coproporphyrinogen (Copro'gen; please note that its generation is indicated in fig. 2) is transported into mitochondria by either peripheral-type benzodiazepine receptors [64] or ABCB6 [65]. Neither mechanisms nor the regulation of the transport of heme from mitochondria to globin polypeptides are known, however it has been proposed that a carrier protein, heme binding protein 1 (gene: *HEBP1*), is involved in this process [66]. CPO = Coprporphyrinogen oxidase; PPO = protoporphyrinogen oxidase.

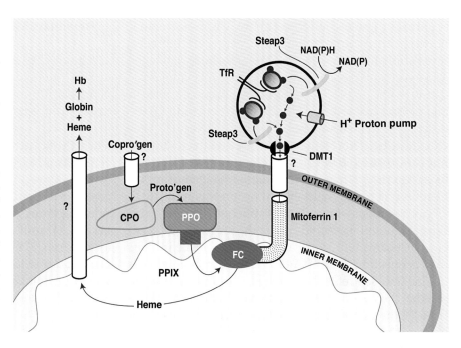

such pool is available for incorporation into SOD2, while the other is not [44]. The substrate of Mtm1/SLC25A39 remains enigmatic.

Amazingly, there are no known mechanisms for the release of any form of iron (e.g. heme, Fe/S peptide/protein, or low-molecular-weight chelate) from mitochondria. One possible explanation for the deposition of iron in mitochondria that are unable to produce Fe/S proteins or heme is that mitochondria may only be capable of releasing 'functional' iron in the form of Fe/S or heme. This idea may be supported by the fact that MFt is capable of sequestering excess iron in these organelles. However, simply increasing the amount of iron in mitochondria has never been shown to induce the presence of the protein in any model. Furthermore, the existence of several CIA factors, including a scaffold for transient Fe/S formation, may suggest that Fe/S can be formed outside mitochondria from an extramitochondrial source of iron. Thus, it cannot be ruled out that a mitochondrial export system for a 'free' form of the metal exists.

Etiology and Pathogenesis of Ring Sideroblast Formation

General Comments

The pathophysiology of ring sideroblast formation in patients with ALAS2 defects and those due to inhibitors of porphyrin biosynthesis (table 1) is likely due to the unique aspects of the regulation of iron metabolism and heme synthesis in erythroid cells [15]. These differences can account for the accumulation of non-heme iron in erythroid mitochondria of sideroblastic anemia patients. In hemoglobin-synthesizing cells, iron is specifically targeted towards mitochondria that avidly take up iron even when the synthesis of PPIX is suppressed [14, 15]. In contrast, non-erythroid cells store iron in excess of metabolic needs within ferritin. Hence, erythroid-specific mechanisms and controls are involved in the transport of iron into mitochondria in erythroid cells. The nature of these processes, including the role of Mfn1, an inner mitochondrial membrane protein which presumably provides Fe^{2+} to FC [34], is poorly understood. Tf-bound iron is used for hemoglobin synthesis [14, 15] with a high degree of efficiency and is targeted into erythroid mitochondria.

Since no intermediate for cytoplasmic iron transport has ever been identified in erythroid cells, the following hypothesis of intracellular iron trafficking in developing red blood cells has been proposed (fig. 4). This model postulates that iron, having been released from Tf in the endosome, is passed directly from protein to protein until it reaches FC [14, 15], which incorporates Fe^{2+} into PPIX [26] in the mitochondrion. Such a transfer bypasses the cytosol, as the movement of iron between proteins could be mediated by a direct interaction of the endosome with the mitochondrion [15, 16]. The results of supporting experiments, conducted using erythroid cells, revealed that: (1) iron, delivered to mitochondria via the Tf-Tf receptor pathway, is unavailable to cytoplasmic chelators [16, 45]; (2) Tf-containing endosomes move to and contact mitochondria in erythroid cells, and (3) endosomal movement is required for iron delivery to mitochondria [16]. These studies also revealed that cytoplasmic iron not bound to Tf is inefficiently utilized for heme biosynthesis and that the endosome-mitochondrion interaction increases chelatable mitochondrial iron [16].

An additional important distinction between erythroid and non-erythroid cells is the presence of a feedback mechanism in which 'uncommitted' heme inhibits iron acquisition from Tf in developing red blood cells [for review, see ref. 15]. Although it is still unresolved whether heme inhibits Tf endocytosis or iron release from Tf, the lack of heme as a negative feedback regulator plays an important role in mitochondrial iron accumulation. In contrast, in non-erythroid cells heme does not inhibit iron acquisition from Tf and iron taken up in excess of metabolic needs accumulates in cytosolic ferritin [9]. It needs to be pointed out that non-heme iron, which accumulates in erythroid mitochondria as a result of inhibited heme synthesis, cannot be released from the organelle unless it is inserted into PPIX [14]. This suggests that mitochondria can release iron only when the metal is in a proper chemical form: in this case, as heme. These considerations provide a framework to the pathogenesis of mitochondrial iron accumulation in erythroblasts of patients with sideroblastic anemia caused by ALAS2 defects as well as those caused by agents inhibiting heme biosynthesis (table 1).

In this context, it is pertinent to mention that the first step in heme biosynthesis (ALA formation, fig. 2) is regulated differently in erythroid and non-erythroid cells. As mentioned above, ALAS2 mRNA contains, in its 5′-UTR, an IRE that is responsible for the translational induction of ALAS2 protein by iron. This means that in erythroid cells the rate-limiting, and thus controlling, step in heme synthesis is not the production of ALA (as is the case in hepatocytes, for example), but the availability of iron. Importantly, heme has no inhibitory effect on either the activity or synthesis of ALAS2 [for review, see ref. 15]. Additionally, whereas heme inhibits the import of ALAS1 into mitochondria, it does not inhibit mitochondrial import of erythroid-specific ALAS [46]. Finally, ALAS2 protein, and not ALAS1, has been found to associate with succinyl coenzyme A synthetase in mitochondria [47].

Hereditary Sideroblastic Anemias

These types of anemias are much less common than primary sideroblastic anemias associated with myelodysplastic syndromes or secondary sideroblastic anemias caused by drugs or toxins (table 1).

X-Linked Sideroblastic Anemia

Of the relatively rare inherited forms, XLSA, caused by mutation in erythroid-specific ALAS2, is the most common [8]. Earlier discussion above suggests that ringed sideroblasts arise in patients with *ALAS2* gene mutations because (1) iron is specifically targeted to erythroid mitochondria; (2) mitochondrial iron cannot be adequately utilized due to lack of PPIX; (3) heme, a negative regulator of iron uptake, is deficient, and (4) iron normally exits erythroid mitochondria after being inserted into PPIX [14, 15].

Shortly after the identification of erythroid-specific ALAS, it became obvious that most XLSA cases were caused by mutations in the *ALAS2* gene [6, 8]. Since the *ALAS2* gene is localized on the X chromosome, it is not surprising that this type of anemia occurs primarily in males. Nevertheless, in some family members, XLSA occurs only in females and is probably lethal in hemizygous male conceptions [8]. Mutations in this gene can cause decreased ALA production by several mechanisms: ALAS2 enzyme exhibits decreased affinity for pyridoxal 5′-phosphate, is unstable, has an abnormal catalytic site, or displays increased susceptibility to mitochondrial proteases [48]. Some of the above observations appear to have important clinical implications, since mutations altering an amino acid situated in the proximity of the pyridoxal 5′-phosphate-binding site exhibit a response to pyridoxine, whereas mutations involving sites of substrate binding, enzyme stability, or folding are refractory to pyridoxine [49].

X-Linked Sideroblastic Anemia with Ataxia

A distinct form of XLSA, XLSA/A, was described in several families; this condition, in contrast to ALAS2-linked disease, is associated with elevated erythrocyte PPIX levels. It was demonstrated that mutations in the *ABCB7* gene are responsible for XLSA/A [39]. The ABCB7 protein is thought to be involved in the transfer of iron sulfur clusters (Fe/S) or an Fe/S precursor from mitochondria to the cytosol [50, for review, see ref. 1]. It is not immediately obvious, however, how the disruption of this export pathway might impede heme biosynthesis. Significantly, microcytic anemia in XLSA/A is accompanied by accumulation of erythrocyte ZnPP [39, 51]. Since the formation of ZnPP requires FC, ABCB7 mutations cannot interfere with the activity of this enzyme. Instead, the loss of function of ABCB7 could somehow diminish the availability of reduced iron required for the assembly of heme from PPIX. Alternatively, reduced levels of cytosolic Fe/S assembly may cause an activation of IRP1 that, in turn, interferes with the translation of ALAS2, resulting in a pathogenesis somewhat akin to the GLRX5 mutation. In any case, in XLSA/A, as is the case in ALAS2-associated sideroblastic anemia, decreased levels of heme likely contribute to the pathogenesis of ring sideroblast formation.

Grx5 Deficiency

Another type of hereditary hypochromic anemia was described in *shiraz* (*sir*) zebrafish mutants [30]. These mutants have a deficiency in Grx5 encoded by a gene (*GLRX5*) whose product is required for Fe/S assembly. This study demonstrated that the loss of the Fe/S in IRP1 blocked ALAS2 translation by binding to the IRE located in the 5′-UTR of *ALAS2* mRNA. Subsequently, a case of GLRX5 deficiency in an anemic male with iron overload and a low number of ringed sideroblasts was reported [4]. As in zebra fish *shiraz* mutants, ferritin levels were low and TfR levels were high in the patient's cells, which can be explained by increased IRP1 binding to IREs in mRNAs of these two proteins. Interestingly, erythroblasts from zebrafish *shiraz* mutants were not found to contain iron-loaded mitochondria.

Refractory Anemia with Ring Sideroblasts

The pathophysiology of RARS, associated with myelodysplastic syndromes, is distinct from the above-discussed XLSA. In patients with RARS, there is no evidence for a decrease in the formation of PPIX; instead, the amount of PPIX is moderately increased [8]. It is conceivable that impaired iron reduction could cause intramitochondrial iron accumulation in patients with myelodysplastic syndromes. The recently discovered ferric reductase, Steap3, is involved in the reduction of Fe^{3+} to Fe^{2+} in endosomes [11]. Based on the model of direct interorganellar transfer of iron [14–16], it can be assumed that there is only one reduction step during the path of iron from endosomes to FC. However, the efficient insertion of ferrous ions into PPIX may still require a reducing environment in mitochondria that would be provided by an uninterrupted respiratory chain. This proposal is compatible with the fact that sideroblastic anemia accompanying Pearson marrow-pancreas syndrome is caused by deletions in mitochondrial DNA genes whose products are involved in electron transport. Indeed, at least some patients with myelodysplasia-associated sideroblastic anemia have been described, whose disease is allegedly caused by acquired mutations in subunits of cytochrome oxidase encoded by mitochondrial DNA [52]. However, a rigorous study failed to find cytochrome oxidase mutations in 10 patients with myelodysplasia-associated sideroblastic anemia [53]. Alternatively, another report provided some evidence that *ABCB7* (see the above discussion on XLSA/A) could be a possible candidate gene for RARS [54].

There is an important message in an early but underappreciated report [55] that in hereditary sideroblastic anemias (highly likely due to ALAS2 defects), ring sideroblasts are found only in late erythroblasts, which synthesize hemoglobin with high speed and efficiency. In contrast, ringed sideroblasts are already found during early erythroid development in patients with 'primary idiopathic sideroblastic anemias'. These findings support the notion that primary acquired sideroblastic anemias (highly likely RARS) are unrelated to a defect in heme biosynthesis, but are due to an iron metabolism alteration that manifests itself in early erythroblasts.

Sideroblastic Anemias Caused by Mitochondrial Defects

Pearson marrow-pancreas syndrome [56] is a mitochondrial cytopathy characterized by sideroblastic anemia, exocrine pancreatic dysfunction, varying degrees of lactic acidosis, and hepatic and renal failure. This disorder is a result of heteroplasmic mitochondrial DNA deletions and relocations.

There are some similarities and some dissimilarities between patients with Pearson marrow-pancreas syndrome and patients with MLASA [57]. In both cases, there are defects in the mitochondrial electron transport chain, likely generating an environment that retards iron access to FC in the reduced form. Both disorders are hereditary but, whereas Pearson's syndrome is caused by large deletions in mitochondrial DNA, MLASA results from a homozygous missense mutation in the nucleus-encoded gene, pseudouridine synthase 1 (*PUS1*). Deficient pseudouridylation of mitochondrial tRNAs has been proposed as an etiology of MLASA [57].

Clinical Features and Therapeutic Strategies

The clinical management of all sideroblastic anemias depends on the severity of anemia. Symptoms of extreme fatigue, exertional angina, or shortness of breath at rest mandate red cell transfusion. The unique clinical presentation and the therapy of specific sideroblastic anemia variants are briefly summarized below; more detailed descriptions are available in the 7 previous editions and upcoming 8th edition of *Williams Hematology,* wherein Ernest Beutler, to whom this issue of *Acta Haematologica* is devoted, wrote and edited many chapters discussing various aspects of sideroblastic anemias [3].

Hereditary Sideroblastic Anemias

Of these uncommon disorders, most are X chromosome linked but some are autosomally inherited. Anemia is usually apparent during the first few months or years of life. However, there are patients in whom microcytic anemia first became evident in the 8th and 9th decade of life and were found to have a microcytic, pyridoxine response anemia apparently related to inherited mutations in the *ALAS2* gene. Splenomegaly may be present. The anemia is microcytic and hypochromic and, in some heterozygous females of the sex-linked form, dimorphism of the red cell population may be evident.

Many patients with hereditary sideroblastic anemia have some response to treatment with pyridoxine in doses of 50–200 mg/day [3, 6]. Responses to pyridoxine may result in an increase in the steady-state hemoglobin level or a decrease in the transfusion requirement, but normalization of the hemoglobin level does not usually occur and the anemia relapses when pyridoxine administration is discontinued.

Iron overloading regularly accompanies this disorder and may be the cause of death [3]. Importantly, iron storage may be enhanced when the mutations of hereditary hemochromatosis are co-inherited. If the anemia is not too severe or if it can be partially corrected by the administration of pyridoxine, phlebotomy may be used to diminish the iron burden. Otherwise it may be advisable to attempt to decrease the amount of body iron by iron chelation.

Marrow transplantation, both ablative and nonmyeloblative, has been used on rare occasions to treat hereditary sideroblastic anemia.

XLSA/A [39, 51] is characterized by neurological impairment typically accompanied by mild anemia. The neurological symptoms include ataxia, dysmetria, dysdiadochokinesis, dysarthria, and intention tremor that are cumulatively referred to as 'spinocerebellar syndrome'. A mild intellectual impairment may also be seen.

Pearson marrow-pancreas syndrome [6, 56], often fatal in infancy or early childhood, is characterized by marrow failure with macrocytic sideroblastic anemia that is typically transfusion dependent. Neutropenia and thrombocytopenia may also be present. There is also an invariable dysfunction in the exocrine pancreas due to fibrosis and acinar atrophy resulting in chronic malabsorption and diarrhea. Lactic acidosis, caused by a defect in oxidative phosphorylation, and other organ dysfunctions, e.g. liver impairment, are also common. The usual causes of death are bacterial sepsis due to neutropenia, metabolic crisis, and hepatic failure. Most patients die in infancy, although there is considerable phenotypic variation, presumably depending upon the number of mitochondria affected and their tissue distribution.

Acquired Sideroblastic Anemias

Primary Sideroblastic Anemias

RARS is a variant of myelodysplastic syndrome, a clonal hematopoietic disorder due to a somatic mutation in a pluripotent hematopoietic stem cell [2]. Its definition and place among myelodysplastic syndromes is found in a recent consensus paper [58].

Anemia is present in >90% of patients. Patients may be asymptomatic or, if anemia is more severe, have the non-specific symptoms of anemia, including pallor, weakness, loss of a sense of well-being, and exertional dyspnea. A small proportion of patients have infections related to severe granulocytopenia or hemorrhage related to severe thrombocytopenia at the time of diagnosis; however, this variant of myelodysplastic syndrome has the lowest probability of symptomatic neutropenia, thrombocytopenia, and acute leukemic transformation among all myelodysplastic syndromes. Hepatomegaly or splenomegaly occurs also rarely in this type of myelodysplastic syndrome [58].

Red cell volume is often increased. The red cells are hypochromic, and commonly have a dimorphic appearance in the blood film, i.e. two populations of red cells can be distinguished: one tends to be relatively normal, whereas the other is anisocytic and hypochromic. Red cell shape abnormalities include oval macrocytes, teardrop, spherical, and fragmented cells. Some patients have slight elliptocytosis and basophilic stippling of red cells [3, 58].

A note regarding the therapy of both hereditary sideroblastic anemia and myelodysplastic syndrome is warranted here. Iron overload, particularly when worsened by repeated blood transfusions, can be an important cause of morbidity and mortality in both conditions. Importantly, anemia in these circumstances can be ameliorated following iron removal [for review, see ref. 8]. This seemingly counterintuitive treatment strategy seems to relieve an inhibition of heme synthesis present due to iron loading in erythroid cells, while not interfering with the delivery of Tf-derived iron for hemoglobin synthesis.

Secondary Sideroblastic Anemias

Lead poisoning (plumbism) has been recognized since antiquity. The ingestion of beverages containing lead leached from highly soluble lead glazes or earthenware containers has been blamed for the decline and fall of the Roman aristocracy and is even now an occasional cause of lead intoxication. Today, lead intoxication in children generally results from ingestion of flaking lead paint or from chewing lead-painted articles. In 1998, 8% of US children were affected. By 2004, the latest date for which data are available, this had dropped to 1% [59]. Lead poisoning is more severe in iron-deficient children, even when adjusted for differing exposure [60].

Red cell life span is slightly decreased and basophilic stippling, resulting from abnormally aggregated ribosomes, is present. Similar morphological abnormalities are also seen in congenital deficiency of pyrimidine 5′-nucleotidase, a red cell enzyme that is also inhibited by lead [61]. However, in chronic lead poisoning, hypochromic microcytic red cells predominate and anemia of lead intoxication is not usually due primarily to hemolysis but rather to marrow suppression [3].

Drugs and chemicals that are most commonly associated with sideroblastic anemia [3] are depicted in table 1.

Many of these are pyridoxine antagonists (i.e. ethanol, isonicotinic acid hydrazide, pyrazinamide, and cycloserine). Thus, it is not surprising that anemia resolves upon administration of pyridoxine, although discontinuation of the offending agent should always be the first step. The red cells are hypochromic, and commonly a dimorphic appearance of the erythrocytes can be recognized in the blood film, i.e. two populations of red cells can be distinguished [3, 58].

Copper Deficiency. In 1974, Dunlop and colleagues described 2 patients with copper deficiency who had extensive bowel surgery and received long-term parenteral hyperalimentation [for review, see ref. 8]. One was also neutropenic. In addition, Gregg et al. [62] described in 2002 a female who, several years after gastroduodenal bypass (Billroth II surgery), developed progressive macrocytic anemia, thrombocytopenia, and leukopenia with numerous ring sideroblasts in the marrow, mimicking refractory anemia with ringed sideroblasts. This patient also had optic neuritis and other neurological abnormalities. The hematologic abnormalities, but not neurological defects, resolved fully with copper therapy, countermanding the need for planned marrow transplantation. A similar hematological picture can be seen with zinc-induced copper deficiency.

Acknowledgments

This work was supported in part by the Canadian Institutes of Health Research (CIHR) to P.P. A.D.S. is supported by a fellowship from the CIHR. D.R.R. thanks the National Health and Medical Research Council of Australia for a Senior Principal Research Fellowship and Project Grants. D.R.R. also gratefully acknowledges a grant from the Muscular Dystrophy Association USA (MDA USA). The authors apologize to those colleagues whose work could not be cited owing to space limitations.

References

1 Napier I, Ponka P, Richardson DR: Iron trafficking in the mitochondrion: novel pathways revealed by disease. Blood 2005;105:1867–1874.
2 Prchal JT, Throckmorton DW, Carroll AJ III, Fuson EW, Gams RA, Prchal JF: A common progenitor for human myeloid and lymphoid cells. Nature 1978;274:590–591.
3 Beutler E: Hereditary and acquired sideroblastic anemias; in Lichtman MA, Kipps TJ, Kaushansky K, Beutler E, Sleigsohn U, Prchal JT (eds): Williams Hematology. New York, McGraw-Hill, 2005, pp 823–828.
4 Camaschella C, Campanella A, De Falco L, Boschetto L, Merlini R, Silvestri L, Levi S, Iolascon A: The human counterpart of zebrafish shiraz shows sideroblastic-like microcytic anemia and iron overload. Blood 2007;110:1353–1358.
5 Guernsey DL, Jiang H, Campagna DR, Evans SC, Ferguson M, Kellogg MD, Lachance M, Matsuoka M, Nightingale M, Rideout A, Saint-Amant L, Schmidt PJ, Orr A, Bottomley SS, Fleming MD, Ludman M, Dyack S, Fernandez CV, Samuels ME: Mutations in mitochondrial carrier family gene SLC25A38 cause nonsyndromic autosomal recessive congenital sideroblastic anemia. Nat Genet 2009;41:651–653.
6 Fleming MD: The genetics of inherited sideroblastic anemias. Semin Hematol 2002;39:270–281.
7 Camaschella C: Recent advances in the understanding of inherited sideroblastic anaemia. Br J Haematol 2008;143:27–38.
8 Bottomley SS: Sideroblastic anemias; in Greer JP, Foerster GM, Paraskevas F, Glader B, Arber DA, Means RT Jr (eds): Wintrobe's Clinical Hematology. Philadelphia, Wolters

Kluwer/Lippincott, Williams & Wilkins, 2009, pp 835–856.

9 Richardson DR, Ponka P: The molecular mechanisms of the metabolism and transport of iron in normal and neoplastic cells. Biochim Biophys Acta 1997;1331:1–40.

10 Wrighting DM, Andrews NC: Iron homeostasis and erythropoiesis. Curr Top Dev Biol 2008;82:141–167.

11 Ohgami RS, Campagna DR, Greer EL, Antiochos B, McDonald A, Chen J, Sharp JJ, Fujiwara Y, Barker JE, Fleming MD: Identification of a ferrireductase required for efficient transferrin-dependent iron uptake in erythroid cells. Nat Genet 2005;37:1264–1269.

12 Mims MP, Prchal JT: Divalent metal transporter 1. Hematology 2005;4:339–345.

13 Breuer W, Shvartsman M, Cabantchik ZI: Intracellular labile iron. Int J Biochem Cell Biol 2008;40:350–354.

14 Richardson DR, Ponka P, Vyoral D: Distribution of iron in reticulocytes after inhibition of heme synthesis with succinylacetone: examination of the intermediates involved in iron metabolism. Blood 1996;87:3477–3488.

15 Ponka P: Tissue-specific regulation of iron metabolism and heme synthesis: distinct control mechanisms in erythroid cells. Blood 1997;89:1–25.

16 Sheftel AD, Zhang AS, Brown C, Shirihai OS, Ponka P: Direct interorganellar transfer of iron from endosome to mitochondrion. Blood 2007;110:125–132.

17 Whitnall M, Rahmanto YS, Sutak R, Xu X, Becker EM, Mikhael MR, Ponka P, Richardson DR: The MCK mouse heart model of Friedreich's ataxia: alterations in iron-regulated proteins and cardiac hypertrophy are limited by iron chelation. Proc Natl Acad Sci USA 2008;105:9757–9762.

18 De Domenico I, McVey Ward D, Kaplan J: Regulation of iron acquisition and storage: consequences for iron-linked disorders. Nat Rev Mol Cell Biol 2008;9:72–81.

19 Muckenthaler MU, Galy B, Hentze MW: Systemic iron homeostasis and the iron-responsive element/iron-regulatory protein (IRE/IRP) regulatory network. Annu Rev Nutr 2008;28:197–213.

20 Meyron-Holtz EG, Ghosh MC, Iwai K, LaVaute T, Brazzolotto X, Berger UV, Land W, Ollivierre-Wilson H, Grinberg A, Love P, Rouault TA: Genetic ablations of iron regulatory proteins 1 and 2 reveal why iron regulatory protein 2 dominates iron homeostasis. EMBO J 2004;23:386–395.

21 Cox TC, Bawden MJ, Martin A, May BK: Human erythroid 5-aminolevulinate synthase: promoter analysis and identification of an iron-responsive element in the mRNA. EMBO J 1991;10:1891–1902.

22 Lok CN, Ponka P: Identification of an erythroid active element in the transferrin receptor gene. J Biol Chem 2000;275:24185–24190.

23 Nemeth E, Ganz T: Regulation of iron metabolism by hepcidin. Annu Rev Nutr 2006;26:323–342.

24 Peslova G, Petrak J, Kuzelova K, Hrdy I, Halada P, Kuchel PW, Soe-Lin S, Ponka P, Sutak R, Becker E, Huang ML, Rahmanto YS, Richardson DR, Vyoral D: Hepcidin, the hormone of iron metabolism, is bound specifically to alpha-2-macroglobulin in blood. Blood 2009;113:6225–6236.

25 Knutson M, Wessling-Resnick M: Iron metabolism in the reticuloendothelial system. Crit Rev Biochem Mol Biol 2003;38:61–88.

26 Ajioka RS, Phillips JD, Kushner JP: Biosynthesis of heme in mammals. Biochim Biophys Acta 2006;1763:723–736.

27 Lill R, Mühlenhoff U: Maturation of iron-sulfur proteins in eukaryotes: mechanisms, connected processes, and diseases. Annu Rev Biochem 2008;77:669–700.

28 Biederbick A, Stehling O, Rosser R, Niggemeyer B, Nakai Y, Elsässer HP, Lill R: Role of human mitochondrial Nfs1 in cytosolic iron-sulfur protein biogenesis and iron regulation. Mol Cell Biol 2006;26:5675–5687.

29 Stehling O, Elsässer HP, Bruckel B, Mühlenhoff U, Lill R: Iron-sulfur protein maturation in human cells: evidence for a function of frataxin. Hum Mol Genet 2004;13:3007–3015.

30 Wingert RA, Galloway JL, Barut B, Foott H, Fraenkel P, Axe JL, Weber GJ, Dooley K, Davidson AJ, Schmid B, Paw BH, Shaw GC, Kingsley P, Palis J, Schubert H, Chen O, Kaplan J, Zon LI: Deficiency of glutaredoxin 5 reveals Fe-S clusters are required for vertebrate haem synthesis. Nature 2005;436:1035–1039.

31 Sheftel AD, Lill R: The power plant of the cell is also a smithy: the emerging role of mitochondria in cellular iron homeostasis. Ann Med 2009;41:82–99.

32 Levi S, Corsi B, Bosisio M, Invernizzi R, Volz A, Sanford D, Arosio P, Drysdale J: A human mitochondrial ferritin encoded by an intronless gene. J Biol Chem 2001;276:24437–24440.

33 Cazzola M, Invernizzi R, Bergamaschi G, Levi S, Corsi B, Travaglino E, Rolandi V, Biasiotto G, Drysdale J, Arosio P: Mitochondrial ferritin expression in erythroid cells from patients with sideroblastic anemia. Blood 2003;101:1996–2000.

34 Shaw GC, Cope JJ, Li L, Corson K, Hersey C, Ackermann GE, Gwynn B, Lambert AJ, Wingert RA, Traver D, Trede NS, Barut BA, Zhou Y, Minet E, Donovan A, Brownlie A, Balzan R, Weiss MJ, Peters LL, Kaplan J, Zon LI, Paw BH: Mitoferrin is essential for erythroid iron assimilation. Nature 2006;440:96–100.

35 Shaw GC, Longer NB, Wang YM, Li LT, Kaplan J, Bloomer JR, Paw BH: Abnormal expression of human mitoferrin (SLC25A37) is associated with a variant of erythropoietic protoporphyria. Blood 2006;108:6A.

36 Shepherd M, Dailey TA, Dailey HA: A new class of [2Fe-2S]-cluster-containing protoporphyrin (IX) ferrochelatases. Biochem J 2006;397:47–52.

37 Whatley SD, Ducamp S, Gouya L, Grandchamp B, Beaumont C, Badminton MN, Elder GH, Holme SA, Anstey AV, Parker M, Corrigall AV, Meissner PN, Hift RJ, Marsden JT, Ma Y, Mieli-Vergani G, Deybach JC, Puy H: C-terminal deletions in the ALAS2 gene lead to gain of function and cause X-linked dominant protoporphyria without anemia or iron overload. Am J Hum Genet 2008;83:408–414.

38 Cavadini P, Biasiotto G, Poli M, Levi S, Verardi R, Zanella I, Derosas M, Ingrassia R, Corrado M, Arosio P: RNA silencing of the mitochondrial ABCB7 transporter in HeLa cells causes an iron-deficient phenotype with mitochondrial iron overload. Blood 2007;109:3552–3559.

39 Bekri S, Kispal G, Lange H, Fitzsimons E, Tolmie J, Lill R, Bishop DF: Human ABC7 transporter: gene structure and mutation causing X-linked sideroblastic anemia with ataxia with disruption of cytosolic iron-sulfur protein maturation. Blood 2000;96:3256–3264.

40 Pondarré C, Antiochos BB, Campagna DR, Clarke SL, Greer EL, Deck KM, McDonald A, Han AP, Medlock A, Kutok JL, Anderson SA, Eisenstein RS, Fleming MD: The mitochondrial ATP-binding cassette transporter Abcb7 is essential in mice and participates in cytosolic iron-sulfur cluster biogenesis. Hum Mol Genet 2006;15:953–964.

41 Pondarré C, Campagna DR, Antiochos B, Sikorski L, Mulhern H, Fleming MD: Abcb7, the gene responsible for X-linked sideroblastic anemia with ataxia, is essential for hematopoiesis. Blood 2007;109:3567–3569.

42 Rademakers LH, Koningsberger JC, Sorber CW, Baart de la Faille H, Van Hattum J, Marx JJ: Accumulation of iron in erythroblasts of patients with erythropoietic protoporphyria. Eur J Clin Invest 1993;23:130–138.

43 Luk E, Carroll M, Baker M, Culotta VC: Manganese activation of superoxide dismutase 2 in Saccharomyces cerevisiae requires MTM1, a member of the mitochondrial carrier family. Proc Natl Acad Sci USA 2003;100:10353–10357.

44 Yang M, Cobine PA, Molik S, Naranuntarat A, Lill R, Winge DR, Culotta VC: The effects of mitochondrial iron homeostasis on cofactor specificity of superoxide dismutase 2. EMBO J 2006;25:1775–1783.

45 Zhang AS, Sheftel AD, Ponka P: Intracellular kinetics of iron in reticulocytes: evidence for endosome involvement in iron targeting to mitochondria. Blood 2005;105:368–375.

46 Munakata H, Sun JY, Yoshida K, Nakatani T, Honda E, Hayakawa S, Furuyama K, Hayashi N: Role of the heme regulatory motif in the heme-mediated inhibition of mitochondrial import of 5-aminolevulinate synthase. J Biochem 2004;136:233–238.

47 Furuyama K, Sassa S: Interaction between succinyl CoA synthetase and the heme-biosynthetic enzyme ALAS-E is disrupted in sideroblastic anemia. J Clin Invest 2000;105:757–764.

48 Furuyama K, Sassa S: Multiple mechanisms for hereditary sideroblastic anemia. Cell Mol Biol (Noisy-le-grand) 2002;48:5–10.

49 Astner I, Schulze JO, van den Heuvel J, Jahn D, Schubert WD, Heinz DW: Crystal structure of 5-aminolevulinate synthase, the first enzyme of heme biosynthesis, and its link to XLSA in humans. EMBO J 2005;24:3166–3177.

50 Lill R, Dutkiewicz R, Elsässer H-P, Hausmann A, Netz DJA, Pierik AJ, Stehling O, Urzica E, Mühlenhoff U: Mechanisms of iron-sulfur protein maturation in mitochondria, cytosol and nucleus of eukaryotes. Biochim Biophys Acta 2006;1763:652–667.

51 Allikmets R, Raskind WH, Hutchinson A, Schueck ND, Dean M, Koeller DM: Mutation of a putative mitochondrial iron transporter gene (ABC7) in X-linked sideroblastic anemia and ataxia (XLSA/A). Hum Mol Genet 1999;8:743–749.

52 Gattermann N: From sideroblastic anemia to the role of mitochondrial DNA mutations in myelodysplastic syndromes. Leuk Res 2000;24:141–151.

53 Shin MG, Kajigaya S, Levin BC, Young NS: Mitochondrial DNA mutations in patients with myelodysplastic syndromes. Blood 2003;101:3118–3125.

54 Boultwood J, Pellagatti A, Nikpour M, Pushkaran B, Fidler C, Cattan H, Littlewood TJ, Malcovati L, Della Porta MG, Jadersten M, Killick S, Giagounidis A, Bowen D, Hellstrom-Lindberg E, Cazzola M, Wainscoat JS: The role of the iron transporter ABCB7 in refractory anemia with ring sideroblasts. PLoS ONE 2008;3:e1970.

55 Hall R, Losowsky MS: The distribution of erythroblast iron in sideroblastic anaemias. Br J Haematol 1966;12:334–340.

56 Pearson HA, Lobel JS, Kocoshis SA, Naiman JL, Windmiller J, Lammi AT, Hoffman R, Marsh JC: A new syndrome of refractory sideroblastic anemia with vacuolization of marrow precursors and exocrine pancreatic dysfunction. J Pediatr 1979;95:976–984.

57 Bykhovskaya Y, Casas K, Mengesha E, Inbal A, Fischel-Ghodsian N: Missense mutation in pseudouridine synthase 1 (PUS1) causes mitochondrial myopathy and sideroblastic anemia (MLASA). Am J Hum Genet 2004;74:1303–1308.

58 Mufti GJ, Bennett JM, Goasguen J, Bain BJ, Baumann I, Brunning R, Cazzola M, Fenaux P, Germing U, Hellstrom-Lindberg E, Jinnai I, Manabe A, Matsuda A, Niemeyer CM, Sanz G, Tomonaga M, Vallespi T, Yoshimi A: Diagnosis and classification of myelodysplastic syndrome: International Working Group on Morphology of myelodysplastic syndrome (IWGM-MDS) consensus proposals for the definition and enumeration of myeloblasts and ring sideroblasts. Haematologica 2008;93:1712–1717.

59 Jones RL, Homa DM, Meyer PA, Brody DJ, Caldwell KL, Pirkle JL, Brown MJ: Trends in blood lead levels and blood lead testing among US children aged 1 to 5 years, 1988–2004. Pediatrics 2009;123:e376–e385.

60 Bradman A, Eskenazi B, Sutton P, Athanasoulis M, Goldman LR: Iron deficiency associated with higher blood lead in children living in contaminated environments. Environ Health Perspect 2001;109:1079–1084.

61 Pagliuca A, Mufti GJ, Baldwin D, Lestas AN, Wallis RM, Bellingham AJ: Lead poisoning: clinical, biochemical, and haematological aspects of a recent outbreak. J Clin Pathol 1990;43:277–281.

62 Gregg XT, Reddy V, Prchal JT: Copper deficiency masquerading as myelodysplastic syndrome. Blood 2002;100:1493–1495.

63 Yu Y, Kalinowski D, Kovacevic Z, Siafakas R, Jansson P, Stefani C, Lovejoy DB, Sharpe PC, Bernhard, PV, Richardson DR: Thiosemicarbazones from the old to new: iron chelators that are more than just ribonucleotide reductase inhibitors. J Med Chem 2009;52:5271–5294.

64 Verma A, Nye JS, Snyder SH: Porphyrins are endogenous ligands for the mitochondrial (peripheral-type) benzodiazepine receptor. Proc Natl Acad Sci USA 1987;84:2256–2260.

65 Krishnamurthy PC, Du G, Fukuda Y, Sun D, Sampath J, Mercer KE, Wang J, Sosa-Pineda B, Murti KG, Schuetz JD: Identification of a mammalian mitochondrial porphyrin transporter. Nature 2006;443:586–589.

66 Jacob BB, Dailey TA, Lianchun X, Dailey HA: Characterization of a human and mouse tetrapyrrole-binding protein. Arch Biochem Biophys 2002;407:196–201.

67 Huang MLH, Becker EM, Whitnall M, Rahmanto YS, Ponka P, Richardson DR: Elucidation of the mechanism of mitochondrial iron loading in Friedreich's ataxia by analysis of a mouse mutant. Proc Natl Acad Sci USA 2009;106:16381–16386.

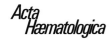

Acta Haematol 2009;122:134–139
DOI: 10.1159/000243797

Published online: November 10, 2009

The Natural History of Untreated *HFE*-Related Hemochromatosis

Paul C. Adams

University Hospital, London, Ont., Canada

Key Words

Arthropathy · C282Y homozygosity · Hemochromatosis · *HFE* · Iron overload · Liver fibrosis · Phlebotomy

Abstract

Hemochromatosis has generally been considered to be a genetic disease in which progressive iron accumulation over many years can lead to cirrhosis of the liver, hepatocellular carcinoma, diabetes, cardiomyopathy, and arthropathy. Iron depletion by phlebotomy has been the recommended therapy although a randomized trial of phlebotomy versus no treatment has never been reported. Since the discovery of the *HFE* gene in 1996, it has been possible to predict the risk of developing iron overload by a simple blood test to detect C282Y homozygotes of the *HFE* gene. The application of the hemochromatosis genetic test in large population studies often initiated to investigate other diseases has provided a fascinating glimpse into the natural history of untreated C282Y homozygotes followed for over 20 years without phlebotomy treatment. These observations are summarized in this review article which raises questions about the need for phlebotomy in all C282Y homozygous patients.

Copyright © 2009 S. Karger AG, Basel

Case History

A 49-year-old postmenopausal Caucasian presents with arthritis in her hands. X-rays of the hands are reported as consistent with hemochromatosis arthropathy [1]. Blood tests at that time demonstrate a serum ferritin of 547 μg/l (normal 15–200 μg/l) and a transferrin saturation of 70% (normal 20–50%). She was offered specialist referral for hemochromatosis at that time but declined. She was seen 7 years later and at that time confirmed to be homozygous for the C282Y mutation of the *HFE* gene. Blood tests without any phlebotomies showed a serum ferritin of 473 μg/l and a transferrin saturation of 61%. There was no clinical evidence of bleeding and serological testing for celiac disease was normal.

Clinical Expression of Hemochromatosis

The classic descriptions of hemochromatosis patients have arisen from referred patients seen in tertiary referral centers. This led to early reports of a high prevalence of clinical symptoms such as cirrhosis of the liver. Even before the description of the *HFE* gene [2], it had been predicted that hemochromatosis could be as common as 1 in 300 in the Caucasian population [3]. There has always been this paradox where experts in the field have empha-

Prof. Paul C. Adams, MD
University Hospital
339 Windermere Road
London, ON N6A 5A5 (Canada)
Tel. +1 519 685 8500, ext. 35375, E-Mail padams@uwo.ca

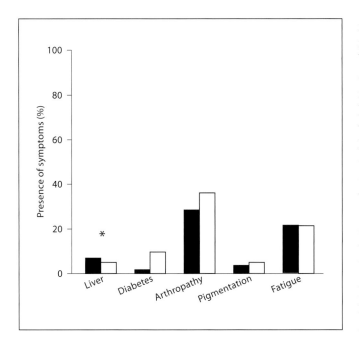

Fig. 1. A comparison of the signs and symptoms of hemochromatosis in 152 screened C282Y homozygotes (■) compared to an age-matched control group (□). The only significant difference between the groups was liver disease (* p < 0.05) [4].

males and no liver biopsies were performed. The authors noted in their abstract that the classical description of bronze diabetes referred to by Sheldon [5] and others occurred in only 1% of patients. This was misinterpreted by many abstract-only readers as the clinical expression of hemochromatosis, and an era of controversy and debate was entered. In the center of this debate was Ernest Beutler, a well-established hematologist from the Scripps Clinic who had made seminal contributions to many other areas of medicine. We soon discovered that Dr. Beutler was a man of great intellect with a logical mind that was a great challenge to debaters around the world. His concepts brought controversy to the field and his dedicated team of researchers complemented their clinical observations by providing ground-breaking studies in molecular genetics. The screening study was criticized for excluding previously diagnosed and treated hemochromatosis patients since they would likely have had more clinical features associated with iron overload. The study did not perform any liver biopsies and may have underestimated the presence of silent hepatic fibrosis. Since the entry point to this study was at a health appraisal clinic it was not entirely unexpected that if you screen healthy people you find healthy people. For investigators in the field of hemochromatosis, there was a concern that these findings would lead to reduced interest and peer-reviewed grant funding, and many of these concerns have proven to be true 8 years after this original publication. Patient support groups also felt bewildered by this report since many of their loved ones had passed away from the complications of iron overload and they did not believe that the adverse effects of iron overload should be minimized.

sized the high prevalence of hemochromatosis whereas established clinicians continued to consider this to be a rare disease. With the discovery of the *HFE* gene, it was possible to study the genotypic prevalence of hemochromatosis and to evaluate the genotypic-phenotypic correlations.

One of the largest trials to address these questions was a screening study at a health appraisal clinic at Kaiser Permanente in San Diego, Calif., USA [4]. In this study, 41,038 healthy participants were tested for ferritin, transferrin saturation and *HFE* testing. A surrogate marker for liver fibrosis was used (collagen IV) and a large age- and gender-matched control group without *HFE* mutations was compared to C282Y homozygotes. The use of a large matched control group was a major advance in the field because it allowed for an estimation of the prevalence of nonspecific symptoms such as fatigue and arthralgias in a similar unaffected population. In this study, there were no significant differences in putative hemochromatosis-related symptoms such as poor general health, diabetes, arthralgias, and pigmentation between 152 C282Y homozygotes and the control group. There was a slight increase in liver disease as assessed by blood tests in the C282Y homozygotes (fig. 1). This was predominantly in

Screening the General Population for Iron Overload

Large-scale population studies screening for iron overload were already in progress in North America [6], Norway [7], France [8], and Australia [9, 10]. The largest of these studies was the HEIRS (Hemochromatosis and Iron Overload Screening) Study [6] which screened 101,168 participants of multi-ethnic origin using *HFE* genotyping, serum ferritin and transferrin saturation. Although the prevalence of the C282Y genotype was 1 in 227 in Caucasians, the prevalence of clinical symptoms was low and mostly indistinguishable from a matched control population [11]. This study did not exclude previously diagnosed cases and was able to analyze their symptoms separately. The Norwegian screening study of 65,238 par-

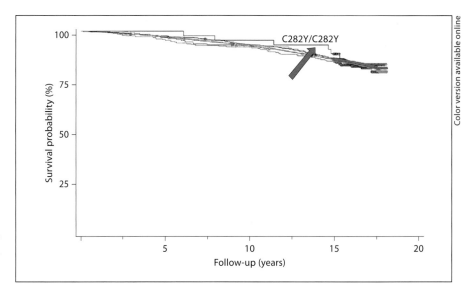

Fig. 2. The actuarial survival of 48 untreated C282Y homozygotes compared to 5 other *HFE* genotypes (C282Y/H63D, H63D/H63D, C282Y/+, H63D/+, and +/+) [14].

ticipants [7] used a phenotype followed by genotype strategy but included data on liver biopsies from 179 participants. The presence of cirrhosis was seen in 5% of the men but none of the women. Clinical symptoms also seemed to be uncommon in their study population [12]. An Australian study that also included liver biopsies documented cirrhosis in 5.6% of their population [10].

Observations on the Natural History of Untreated C282Y Homozygotes

Clinical trials of phlebotomy therapy including a no-treatment arm were considered to be unethical because of the published reports of the beneficial effects of iron depletion on symptoms and survival. A number of population studies that had been initiated for other reasons such as cardiovascular diseases were able to do C282Y genotyping on their patient cohorts many years after the studies had begun. This resulted in the discovery of C282Y homozygotes that had been under observation for many years. They were untreated for hemochromatosis because they were unaware of their risk of iron overload predicted by their genotype.

In the Busselton study in Western Australia, volunteers from a town are followed and assessed serially for many years to study a wide variety of health problems. In the 3,011 study participants, data became available on 16 homozygotes that had been followed for 17 years [13]. In some of these participants, serum ferritin was not rising, raising the possibility that progressive iron accumulation

in C282Y homozygotes is not inevitable. This hypothesis was confirmed in the Copenhagen Heart Study [14] in which 23 homozygotes were followed for 25 years. The ARIC (Atherosclerosis Research in Communities) study was able to identify 44 C282Y homozygotes followed for 17 years and there was no difference in survival between the C282Y homozygotes and the 5 other *HFE* genotypes (fig. 2) [15]. However, liver disease was detected in 11% of these homozygotes and 2 of these homozygotes died from liver cancer. Another large study in Melbourne, Australia, was able to follow 203 homozygotes for 12 years without phlebotomy. In this study, it was once again demonstrated that many C282Y homozygotes do not have a rising serum ferritin over time. Population models were presented to predict the risk of developing iron overload based on the presenting transferrin saturation and ferritin. It was also noted in this study that many postmenopausal females did not demonstrate a rising ferritin over the observation period [16]. This study emphasized that there is still a significant iron-related morbidity seen in 28% of the men and 1% of the women [10].

Do All C282Y Homozygotes Require Phlebotomy Therapy?

Iron depletion by phlebotomy has been widely advocated for C282Y homozygotes with an elevated serum ferritin (in males >300 μg/l and in females >200 μg/l) [17]. This recommendation was not based on the presence of symptoms at these thresholds. It was assumed that a

C282Y homozygote with an elevated ferritin is on a trajectory of progressive iron overload and phlebotomy could prophylactically prevent the anticipated complications. If many homozygotes are not progressing, why would they need phlebotomy therapy? A serum ferritin of >1,000 μg/l has been associated with significant liver disease and is a better-established threshold for the initiation of phlebotomy [18]. This led some groups to recommend using a serum ferritin of >1,000 μg/l as the preferred screening test for hemochromatosis in the general population [19]. The diagnosis could be confirmed by genetic testing and there may be some medical benefit to the other participants with elevated ferritin who may be found to have other infectious, inflammatory, metabolic, or neoplastic conditions.

Many physicians and patients have expressed their concerns that any excess iron is potentially deleterious to health and why wait until liver fibrosis may have started to offer phlebotomy. Some patients describe a positive health state after each phlebotomy and in some cases blood removed by phlebotomy can be used for blood donation. Liver fibrosis is potentially reversible by phlebotomy and it is uncommon in C282Y homozygotes with a normal AST and ALT [20]. If phlebotomy treatment was to be selectively offered to C282Y homozygotes, how could the risk of iron accumulation be predicted? An elevated transferrin saturation has predictive value, although the test has considerable biological variability. A ferritin approaching 1,000 μg/l also predicts a patient that may reach that threshold. A plot of serum ferritin in an untreated C282Y homozygote over a period of 6 months or longer may be a method of predicting progressive iron overload. The rising slopes of ferritin which are available from the previously mentioned studies have been shown to vary widely, and may not rise in a linear pattern [16]. These observations that many untreated C282Y homozygotes are not demonstrating progressive iron overload may open the door for a randomized study of phlebotomy versus no phlebotomy in patients that present with a serum ferritin <1,000 μg/l. If a patient with a ferritin <1,000 μg/l is phlebotomy intolerant (no venous access, phlebitis, or vasovagal events), a trial of observation without treatment may be a preferable option to oral iron chelation (cost/side effects) or indwelling intravenous catheters (thrombosis, infection, or anticoagulation). The debate about phlebotomy therapy also includes issues surrounding the endpoints of phlebotomy therapy and the need for maintenance therapy. The current recommendations to continue iron depletion until the serum ferritin is low (20–50 μg/l) are not evidence based. It was believed that many patients should be treated to a low ferritin since it would then allow them time to slowly reaccumulate iron through the normal ferritin range. If they are not destined to re-accumulate iron [21], they may have been overtreated. These concepts also apply to maintenance phlebotomy which also has the potential to increase intestinal iron absorption. Some physicians advocate treatment to a low serum ferritin to be able to normalize the transferrin saturation. This is based on experimental animal studies which have suggested that elevations in non-transferrin-bound iron can be toxic to cells. There is no evidence that demonstrates that iron depletion to a serum ferritin in the normal range is inferior to iron depletion to a serum ferritin of 20 μg/l. Excess iron depletion can turn an asymptomatic patient into a symptomatic patient and should be discouraged. Many of the patient support groups have become militant about reaching these low iron targets.

Pathogenesis of Variable Biochemical and Clinical Expression in Hemochromatosis

In the classic monograph of Sheldon [5] in 1935 which described over 300 clinical cases of hemochromatosis, he concluded that hemochromatosis was a disease worthy of the fullest possible study because at that moment the study of the metallic constituents of the cell was shrouded in mystery. In 1996, the HFE gene was discovered, but the function of the HFE protein and the pathogenesis of the disease have not been fully elucidated. Our current understanding is that patients with hemochromatosis and iron overload may have a defect in iron sensing possibly within the liver. In a normal human, the HFE protein is bound to the transferrin receptor (TfR1) at the surface of the cell membrane. As excess transferrin-bound iron is sensed in the blood, the HFE protein shifts to another transferrin receptor (TfR2) which is linked to another membrane complex of proteins including bone morphogenic protein (BMP6) and hemojuvelin. This complex activates the production of intracellular hepcidin through a pathway involving the phosphorylation of the intracellular Smad proteins. In C282Y homozygotes, there is a conformational change in the HFE protein which leads to a defective trafficking of the HFE protein to the cell surface. The net result is a low circulating serum hepcidin which increases dietary intestinal iron absorption. This low hepcidin persists even as iron accumulates because of this defect in iron sensing [22].

One of the great mysteries of hemochromatosis is the wide variability in clinical expression of the disease, and a tool to predict the natural history of an individual C282Y homozygote based on a biochemical or genetic profile would be a significant advance. Some of the known factors which may affect expression include age, gender, alcohol, and obesity. It has been difficult to demonstrate a strong effect of dietary iron, and there have been reports on effects of tea consumption and gastric-acid-suppressing medications to suppress iron absorption. There has been interest in the possibility of co-modifying genes although pedigrees of non-expressing C282Y homozygotes have rarely been reported. Many investigators have studied polymorphisms in other known iron genes such as TfR2, hepcidin, hemojuvelin, and ferroportin. Rare cases have been reported with multiple genetic mutations but the 'missing link' has not been established at this time. A novel theory was proposed that the C282Y mutation in the *HFE* gene is the modifying gene and the true hemochromatosis gene is yet to be discovered [23–28].

Conclusion

These observations on the natural history of untreated C282Y homozygotes should not lead us to forget that there remains a small number of male C282Y homozygotes that may present with advanced cirrhosis or hepatocellular carcinoma. The recommendations against population screening by many public health groups [29] is not a recommendation against appropriate treatment in referred patients. The challenge in the future will be the ability to select the ideal candidates for iron depletion therapy.

References

1 Adams PC, Barton JC: Haemochromatosis. Lancet 2007;370:1855–1860.
2 Feder JN, Gnirke A, Thomas W, Tsuchihashi Z, Ruddy DA, Basava A, Dormishian F, Domingo R Jr, Ellis MC, Fullan A, Hinton LM, Jones NL, Kimmel BE, Kronmal GS, Lauer P, Lee VK, Loeb DB, Mapa FA, McClelland E, Meyer NC, Mintier GA, Moeller N, Moore T, Morikang E, Prass CE, Quintana L, Starnes SM, Schatzman RC, Brunke KJ, Drayna DT, Risch NJ, Bacon BR, Wolff RK: A novel MHC class I-like gene is mutated in patients with hereditary hemochromatosis. Nat Genet 1996;13:399–408.
3 Edwards CQ, Griffen LM, Goldgar D, Drummond C, Skolnick MH, Kushner JP: Prevalence of hemochromatosis among 11,065 presumably healthy blood donors. N Engl J Med 1988;318:1355–1362.
4 Beutler E, Felitti V, Koziol J, Ho N, Gelbart T: Penetrance of the 845G→A (C282Y) HFE hereditary haemochromatosis mutation in the USA. Lancet 2002;359:211–218.
5 Sheldon JH: Haemochromatosis. Oxford, Oxford Medical Publications, 1935, pp 164–340.
6 Adams PC, Reboussin DM, Barton JC, McLaren CE, Eckfeldt JH, McLaren GD, Dawkins FW, Acton RT, Harris EL, Gordeuk VR, Leiendecker-Foster C, Speechley M, Snively BM, Holup JL, Thomson E, Sholinsky P: Hemochromatosis and iron-overload screening in a racially diverse population. N Eng J Med 2005;352:1769–1778.

7 Asberg A, Hveem K, Thorstensen K, Ellekjaer E, Kannelonning K, Fjosne U, Halvorsen TB, Smethurst HB, Sagen E, Bjerve KS: Screening for hemochromatosis – high prevalence and low morbidity in an unselected population of 65,238 persons. Scand J Gastroenterol 2001;36:1108–1115.
8 Deugnier Y, Jouanolle A, Chaperon J, Moirand R, Pithois C, Meyer J, Pouchard M, Lafraise B, Brigand A, Caserio-Schoenemann C, Mosser J, Adams P, Le Gall JY, David V: Gender-specific phenotypic expression and screening strategies in C282Y-linked haemochromatosis. Br J Haematol 2002;118:1170–1178.
9 Delatycki M, Allen K, Nisselle A, Collins V, Metcalfe S, du Sart D, Halliday J, Aitken MA, Macciocca I, Hill V, Wakefield A, Ritchie A, Gason AA, Nicoll AJ, Powell LW, Williamson R: Use of community genetic screening to prevent HFE-associated hereditary haemochromatosis. Lancet 2005;366:314–316.
10 Powell LW, Dixon JL, Ramm GA, Anderson GJ, Subramanian VN, Hewett DG, Searle JW, Fletcher LM, Crawford DH, Rodgers H, Allen KJ, Cavanaugh JA, Bassett ML: Screening for hemochromatosis in asymptomatic subjects with or without a family history. Arch Intern Med 2006;166:294–301.
11 McLaren GD, McLaren CE, Adams PC, Barton JC, Reboussin DM, Gordeuk VR, Acton RT, Harris EL, Speechley MR, Sholinsky P, Dawkins FW, Snively BM, Vogt TM, Eckfeldt JH, Hemochromatosis and Iron Overload Screen (HEIRS) Study Research Investigators: Clinical manifestations of hemochromatosis in *HFE* C282Y homozygotes identified by screening. Can J Gastroenterol 2008;22:923–930.

12 Asberg A, Hveem K, Kruger O, Bjerve K: Persons with screening-detected haemochromatosis: as healthy as the general population? Scand J Gastroenterol 2002;37:719–724.
13 Olynyk J, Hagan S, Cullen D, Beilby J, Whittall D: Evolution of untreated hereditary hemochromatosis in the Busselton population: a 17-year study. Mayo Clin Proc 2004;79:309–313.
14 Andersen RV, Tybjaerg-Hansen A, Appleyard M, Birgens H, Nordestgaard BG: Hemochromatosis mutations in the general population: iron overload progression rate. Blood 2004;103:2914–2919.
15 Pankow JS, Boerwinkle E, Adams PC, Guallar E, Leiendecker-Foster C, Rogowski J, Eckfeldt JH: HFE C282Y homozygotes have reduced low-density lipoprotein cholesterol: the Atherosclerosis Risk in Communities (ARIC) Study. Transl Res 2008;152:3–10.
16 Gurrin LC, Osborne NJ, Constantine CC, McLaren CE, English DR, Gertig DM, Delatycki MB, Southey MC, Hopper JL, Giles GG, Anderson GJ, Olynyk JK, Powell LW, Allen KJ: The natural history of serum iron indices for HFE C282Y homozygosity associated with hereditary hemochromatosis. Gastroenterology 2008;135:1945–1952.
17 Barton J, McDonnell S, Adams PC, Brissot P, Powell L, Edwards C, Cook J, Kowdley K: Management of hemochromatosis. Ann Intern Med 1998;129:932–939.
18 Beaton M, Guyader D, Deugnier Y, Moirand R, Chakrabarti S, Adams P: Non-invasive prediction of cirrhosis in C282Y-linked hemochromatosis. Hepatology 2002;36:673–678.

19 Waalen J, Felitti VJ, Gelbart T, Beutler E: Screening for hemochromatosis by measuring ferritin levels: a more effective approach. Blood 2008;111:3373–3376.

20 Beaton M, Adams PC: Assessment of silent liver fibrosis in hemochromatosis C282Y homozygotes with normal transaminase levels. Clin Gastroenterol Hepatol 2008;6:713–714.

21 Adams PC, Kertesz AE, Valberg LS: Rate of iron reaccumulation following iron depletion in hereditary hemochromatosis. Implications for venesection therapy. J Clin Gastroenterol 1993;16:207–210.

22 Ganz T: Iron homeostasis: fitting the puzzle pieces together. Cell Metab 2008;7:288–90.

23 Beutler E: Natural history of hemochromatosis. Mayo Clin Proc 2004;79:305–306.

24 Beutler E: The HFE Cys282Tyr mutation as a necessary but not sufficient cause of clinical hereditary hemochromatosis. Blood 2003; 101:3347–3350.

25 Lee PL, Barton JC, Brandhagen D, Beutler E: Hemojuvelin (HJV) mutations in persons of European, African-American and Asian ancestry with adult onset haemochromatosis. Br J Haematol 2004;127:224–229.

26 Truksa J, Peng H, Lee P, Beutler E: Bone morphogenetic proteins 2, 4, and 9 stimulate murine hepcidin 1 expression independently of Hfe, transferrin receptor 2 (Tfr2), and IL-6. Proc Natl Acad Sci USA 2006;103:10289–10293.

27 Beutler E, Barton J, Felitti V, Gelbart T, West C, Lee P, Lee PL, Waalen J, Vulpe C: Ferroportin 1 (SCL40A1) variant associated with iron overload in African-Americans. Blood Cells Mol Dis 2003;31:305–309.

28 Lee P, Gelbart T, West C, Halloran C, Felitti V, Beutler E: A study of genes that may modulate the expression of hereditary hemochromatosis: transferrin receptor-1, ferroportin, ceruloplasmin, ferritin light and heavy chains, iron regulatory proteins (IRP)-1 and -2, and hepcidin. Blood Cells Mol Dis 2001;27:783–802.

29 Whitlock E, Garlitz B, Harris EL, Beil TL, Smith PR: Screening for hereditary hemochromatosis: a systematic review for the U.S. Preventive Services Task Force. Ann Intern Med 2006;145:209–223.

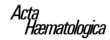

Acta Haematol 2009;122:140–145
DOI: 10.1159/000243798

Published online: November 10, 2009

Rare Types of Genetic Hemochromatosis

Clara Camaschella   Erika Poggiali

Vita-Salute University and San Raffaele Scientific Institute, Milan, Italy

Key Words

Iron · Hemochromatosis · Hepcidin · Ferroportin · Hemojuvelin

Abstract

Most types of genetic hemochromatosis are due to mutations in the *HFE* gene, although similar iron overload and organ damage can also result from mutations in genes other than *HFE* in rare types of hemochromatosis. Non-*HFE* hemochromatoses have been divided into two subgroups with distinctive features. The first includes juvenile and *TFR2*-related hemochromatoses that, similar to *HFE* hemochromatosis, show recessive inheritance, increased transferrin saturation, iron storage in hepatocytes and responsiveness to phlebotomy. Disorders in this subgroup, although differing regarding the severity of iron overload and/or the age at presentation, are all either due to hepcidin deficiency or to the inability to increase hepcidin levels according to iron stores. The second subgroup of hemochromatosis is caused by autosomal dominant mutations in the *SLC40A1* gene encoding the iron exporter ferroportin with distinctive features. Iron loading of Kupffer cells and normal transferrin saturation characterize the so-called 'ferroportin disease'. In contrast, few mutations in *SLC40A1* that cause hepcidin resistance lead to a hemochromatosis-like phenotype with dominant inheritance. The precise diagnosis of the genetic type of hemochromatosis is relevant for the follow-up, treatment, and for family counseling.

Copyright © 2009 S. Karger AG, Basel

Introduction

Genetic hemochromatosis includes a heterogeneous group of disorders, which is related to hepcidin deficiency, leading to iron overload and eventually organ failure caused by inappropriately high intestinal iron absorption. In the vast majority of patients, hemochromatosis is associated with homozygosity for the C282Y mutation in the *HFE* gene. In the remaining cases, often referred to as 'non-*HFE* hemochromatosis', mutations occur in genes encoding different proteins involved in the pathway of systemic iron regulation [1]. In juvenile or type II hemochromatosis, mutations occur either in hemojuvelin *(HJV* or *HFE2)-* or in hepcidin *(HAMP)*-encoding genes; in type III hemochromatosis they affect transferrin receptor 2 *(TFR2)*, and in type IV hemochromatosis mutations occur in *SLC40A1* encoding the iron exporter ferroportin (table 1). These disorders are not restricted to specific racial or ethnic groups, occur worldwide, and account for most hereditary hemochromatoses unlinked to the *HFE* gene. Whether mutations in other genes may cause hemochromatosis remains to be demonstrated.

Non-*HFE* hemochromatosis is uncommon, but studies on these rare disorders have significantly contributed to improving our understanding of the biological mechanisms regulating systemic iron homeostasis [2]. The discovery that juvenile hemochromatosis is due to mutations in either hepcidin or hemojuvelin provided more insight into signal transduction that regulates hepcidin transcription by bone morphogenetic proteins (BMPs) and the molecular mechanisms of hepcidin activation/ inhibition in conditions of iron overload and deficiency,

KARGER

Fax +41 61 306 12 34
E-Mail karger@karger.ch
www.karger.com

© 2009 S. Karger AG, Basel
0001–5792/09/1223–0140$26.00/0

Accessible online at:
www.karger.com/aha

Prof. Clara Camaschella
Università Vita-Salute San Raffaele
Via Olgettina 60
IT–20132 Milano (Italy)
Tel. +39 02 2643 7782, Fax +39 02 2643 2640, E-Mail clara.camaschella@hsr.it

Table 1. Genetic forms of hemochromatosis not associated with *HFE* mutations

Hemochromatosis type	OMIM No.	Chr.	Gene	Murine models	Mechanism	Phenotype
IIA: juvenile	602390	1q	HFE2	Hamp–/–	low/absent hepcidin	severe early onset, high TS, iron in hepatocytes
IIB: juvenile	602390	19	HAMP	Hjv–/–	reduced Hamp activation	severe early onset, high TS, iron in hepatocytes
III	604250	7q	TFR2	Tfr2–/– $Tfr2^{Y245X/Y245X}$ Tfr2 LC	impaired iron sensor?	early onset, high TS iron in hepatocytes
IV: hemochroma-tosis like	606069	2q	SLC40A1		hepcidin resistance	high TS, iron in hepatocytes
IV: ferroportin disease	606069	2q	SLC40A1	flatiron	reduced macrophage iron export	normal TS, iron in macrophages

OMIM = Online mendelian inheritance in men (http://www.ncbi.nlm.nih.gov/sites/entrez); Chr. = chromosome; TS = transferrin saturation; *Tfr2 LC* = liver conditional knockout mouse.

respectively. The identification of *TFR2* as the gene of hemochromatosis type III and its association with *HFE* paved the way for the development of the model of the hepatic iron sensor. The different phenotypes associated with ferroportin mutations have stimulated research on the function of the different domains of the molecule.

Juvenile or Type II Hemochromatosis

Juvenile hemochromatosis is a rare recessive disorder due to mutations in either *HJV* encoding hemojuvelin (type IIA) or *HAMP* encoding hepcidin (type IIB; table 1). Mutations in either gene produce a similar phenotype. Elevated serum iron indices and iron deposition in parenchymal cells present earlier than in *HFE* hemochromatosis, even in the 1st decade of life. The iron overload is severe and clinical symptoms usually develop before 30 years [3].

Molecular Genetics

Soon after the discovery of the *HFE* gene, it became clear that juvenile hemochromatosis was unrelated to *HFE* mutations. Linkage to chromosome 6 was excluded in consanguineous and multiplex families, in which different chromosome 6 haplotypes segregated in the affected individuals. The first type of juvenile hemochromatosis characterized at the molecular level was type IIB: homozygous causal mutations in the *HAMP* gene, which

encodes the liver peptide hepcidin, were identified in two families [4]. At that time, the role of hepcidin as the key iron regulator was known in mice. Hepcidin, a peptide synthesized in the liver, responds to iron overload and regulates the surface expression of the cellular iron exporter ferroportin [5]. Few families with *HAMP* mutations have been reported and most have a juvenile phenotype. Mutated alleles are either 'null' or affect the invariable cysteines of the protein. A mutation repeatedly found in Portuguese families –25G→A in the 5'>untranslated region creates a new ATG initiation codon out of frame that in vitro prevents normal transcription from the original ATG. A mutation (R59G) which affects the consensus sequence for the proconvertase-mediated cleavage of the active peptide from the propeptide was documented in 2 adult patients [Camaschella and Arosio, unpubl. results] with severe disorders. It has not been established whether residual hepcidin activity persists in these cases.

Most juvenile-onset cases map to chromosome 1q21, where the gene that encodes hemojuvelin (*HFE2* or *HJV*) is localized [6]. Clustering of type IIA hemochromatosis is present in Greece [6], Italy [7], and in the genetically isolated French-Canadian region of Saguenay-Lac-Saint-Jean [7]. Multiple mutations affect the *HJV* gene, resulting in either truncated proteins or proteins with amino acid substitutions [6–8]. Homozygosity for G320V accounts for most cases in individuals of European origin. At variance with *HFE* mutations reported only in Caucasians, *HJV* mutations have been found in Japan in middle-aged severe cases [9] and on the Indian subcontinent in young patients not presenting cardiac disease [10]. It is likely that different genetic modifiers are present in cases of different racial background.

Pathophysiology

At the time of its discovery, the role of HJV in iron metabolism was ambiguous, although the extremely low levels of hepcidin found in patients with *HJV* mutations suggested a function upstream of hepcidin. HJV is a member of the repulsive guidance molecules (RGM) family and is predominantly expressed by hepatocytes, and cardiac and skeletal muscle cells. As other RGMs, HJV is a coreceptor for BMPs that activate hepcidin signaling through SMAD proteins in hepatocytes [11], thereby clarifying why both *HAMP* and *HJV* mutations lead to the same phenotype. HJV is expressed on the basal membrane of murine periportal hepatocytes [12]. Several mutations abrogate HJV cell surface expression and its function as BMP coreceptor that blocks the signaling mechanism of hepcidin activation. Amino acid changes in specific domains likely produce dysfunctional proteins unable to contribute to the surface hepcidin activation complex. The function of HJV in other organs remains to be elucidated.

Mice models of the disease ($Hjv^{-/-}$ and $Hamp^{-/-}$) reproduce the severity of iron loading seen in young patients. They confirm that HJV is critical for the regulation of iron homeostasis and hepcidin transcription. The strong reduction in hepcidin transcription in $Hjv^{-/-}$ mice [12] and the lack of response to iron are associated with ferroportin hyperactivity in enterocytes and macrophages and increased plasma iron. Recent studies show that BMP6 is the endogenous regulator of hepcidin [13] and the phenotype of $Bmp6^{-/-}$ mice indicated *BMP6* as a potential candidate gene for undiagnosed forms of juvenile hemochromatosis.

Clinical Features

Juvenile hemochromatosis is the most severe form of hemochromatosis: iron absorption in the gut is remarkably enhanced compared with *HFE* hemochromatosis; parenchymal iron accumulation occurs rapidly, and clinical manifestations appear at a younger age in both sexes. The disease shows all the features of *HFE* hemochromatosis, e.g. hypogonadotropic hypogonadism, liver cirrhosis, diabetes mellitus, arthropathy, and cardiomyopathy, but all complications are anticipated and more severe [3]. Abdominal pain is the main symptom in children and hypogonadism the most evident in young individuals, whereas refractory heart failure or major arrhythmias are the cause of death in the absence of treatment [3]. Diagnosis of juvenile hemochromatosis is based upon age at presentation, clinical complications, severity of iron overload, and genetic testing. Transferrin saturation is usually 100% or higher, serum ferritin is strikingly elevated, and genetic tests for *HFE* mutations are negative. Second-level tests may identify the mutation(s) in *HJV* or *HAMP* genes. Genetic testing is worthwhile even in children because of the early expression of the disease and the possibility of prevention. Due to the severity of the iron burden, it is advisable to assess liver (and cardiac) iron even in asymptomatic patients, using either invasive (liver biopsy and liver iron concentration determination) or noninvasive methods based on magnetic resonance imaging.

Treatment

Similar to *HFE*-related hemochromatosis, treatment of juvenile hemochromatosis is based on regular and intensive phlebotomy protocols until iron depletion is accomplished (serum ferritin <50 ng/ml and transferrin saturation <30%). It should be emphasized that, similar to type I hemochromatosis, early iron depletion by phlebotomy prevents organ damage and all disease manifestations [3]. Phlebotomy should be performed even in children to prevent liver fibrosis. In the presence of congestive heart failure, iron chelators are indicated not only to reduce the iron burden but also the production of reactive oxygen species. In some cases, small-volume phlebotomy may be combined with iron chelators, such as subcutaneous deferoxamine infusions. A single patient with type II disease and severe heart failure was successfully treated with a combination of deferoxamine and deferiprone [14]. Once iron depletion is achieved, monthly phlebotomy usually maintains serum iron parameters within the normal range. Selected cases with advanced cardiac disease are candidates for heart transplantation. Analogous to *HFE* hemochromatosis, diabetes and hypopituitarism are irreversible and require lifelong hormone replacement. Arthritis is likewise unresponsive to phlebotomy. Estrogen-progesterone treatment restores menstrual cycles in females with secondary amenorrhea, also contributing to iron depletion. Gonadotropins are used to induce pregnancy in iron-depleted women. Analogous to all forms of hemochromatosis, alcohol consumption should be restricted and ingestion of iron-containing preparations avoided.

Recently, it has been reported that treatment with the oral chelator deferasirox is able to effectively reduce liver, heart, and partially (on long-term treatment) pancreatic iron burden in $Hjv^{-/-}$ mice [15]. Whether this drug might become an option for patients requires further studies.

TFR2-Related (Type III) Hemochromatosis

This was the second genetic type of hemochromatosis recognized after the cloning of the *HFE* gene [15] and is caused by mutations in *TFR2*. Type III hemochromatosis is a rare condition identified in few families worldwide [for review, see ref. 16].

Molecular Genetics
The *TFR2* gene encodes a transmembrane protein member of the transferrin receptor (TFRC) family, with moderate homology to TFR1. TFR2 is highly expressed in the liver, where it contributes to maintaining iron homeostasis. The first patients described were homozygous for a nonsense mutation (Y250X) that causes a truncated protein [17]. Other mutations, spread along the entire sequence, have been identified in Europe and Japan [10].

Pathogenesis
HFE is able to bind TFR1 in the presence of apotransferrin and to TFR2 when transferrin is iron loaded. A current functional model suggests that TFR2 coupled with HFE in the presence of diferric transferrin is the likely sensor of iron levels and may regulate hepcidin production, although the molecular mechanisms remain unknown.

Several animal models of *Tfr2* hemochromatosis are available: mice$^{Y245X/Y245X18}$ homozygote for the mutation orthologous to Y250X present in patients [17] have liver iron overload similar to that shown by the *Tfr2$^{-/-}$* [18] and by the liver-specific *Tfr2*-deficient mice [19]. In both patients with type III hemochromatosis and *Tfr2*-deficient mice, hepcidin levels are low and inappropriate to iron stores [19, 20]. However, how TFR2 increases hepcidin transcription remains unclear.

Clinical Features
Type III hemochromatosis is less severe than juvenile hemochromatosis and more similar to *HFE* hemochromatosis, although age at onset may be anticipated (table 1). Clinical features include abnormal liver function tests, cirrhosis, arthritis, diabetes, hypogonadism, cardiomyopathy, and skin pigmentation [16]. Type III hemochromatosis shows variable degrees of iron overload even within the same family, ranging from asymptomatic cases to patients with several iron-related complications [16]. Some patients have iron overload early in life [16]. Iron deposition occurs in periportal hepatocytes as in *HFE* hemochromatosis [21]. Although TFR2 is expressed in peripheral blood mononuclear cells and bone marrow, no red cell abnormalities are observed in the patients. Urinary hepcidin levels were low in the few patients studied [20].

Treatment
Experience in patients with this type of hemochromatosis is limited. Patients are usually treated with the same phlebotomy protocol used for *HFE*-related hemochromatosis. All its complications can be prevented by correct treatment. Patients tolerate phlebotomy well without developing anemia.

Type IV Hemochromatosis (Ferroportin Disease)

Type IV is an autosomal dominant hemochromatosis due to mutations in the cellular iron exporter ferroportin. Compared with the other hemochromatosis forms, type IV has distinct genetic, biochemical, histological, and clinical features that deserve the definition of 'ferroportin disease' [1]. The typical ferroportin disease has iron stored in Kupffer cells instead of hepatocytes and normal/low transferrin saturation levels. However, patients with 'atypical' ferroportin disease have a phenotype indistinguishable from classic hemochromatosis (table 1). Functional studies have shown that this difference is mostly related to the mutation type.

Molecular Genetics
Ferroportin is a ubiquitous multiple-transmembrane-domain protein, which is highly expressed in enterocytes, macrophages, and syncytiotrophoblasts, where it exports iron. Its surface expression and activity are controlled by hepcidin [4]. The first mutations N144H and A77D were identified in large families from The Netherlands [22] and Italy [23], respectively. A number of *missense* mutations, often restricted to single families, associated with variable phenotypes [2] have been established in Europeans and Asians. They are all rare, except the valine deletion at position 162 (V162del), which has repeatedly been reported. *Nonsense* mutations have never been described. The polymorphic change Q284H is a highly frequent finding in African and African-Americans and therefore potential involvement in African iron overload has been assumed, but the association remains equivocal [24].

Pathogenesis
Mutations in ferroportin may not only affect its presentation on the plasma membrane, but also its ability to transport iron, to bind hepcidin, or to be internalized [25]. For this reason, type IV hemochromatosis is convenient-

ly classified in two forms according to the phenotype and the mutation type. In the typical 'ferroportin disease', *loss-of-function* mutations – such as A77D and V162del – lead to decreased surface expression of the mutant protein, decreased iron export, abnormal retention of iron in macrophages [26], a reduced plasma iron pool, and iron-restricted erythropoiesis. Whether these mutations cause haploinsufficiency or have a dominant negative effect has been a matter of debate, but recent data favor the dominant negative mechanism [27]. Other ferroportin mutations, such as the substitution of either serine or tyrosine for cysteine at position 326, result in ferroportin molecules that correctly localize to the plasma membrane and export iron normally. However, they are unable to bind hepcidin, leading to a *gain-of-function* phenotype, because the permanently 'switched-on' ferroportin increases iron export to the circulation. Other mutations as N144 and Y64 affect the ability of hepcidin to internalize the hepcidin-ferroportin complex [25]. The phenotype of these 'hepcidin-resistant' forms is similar to the hepcidin-deficient phenotype of classic hemochromatosis.

The essential role of ferroportin for maternal-fetal iron transfer explains why type IV hemochromatosis is autosomal dominant. Mice heterozygous for the ferroportin constitutive deletion do not show any abnormality, suggesting that haploinsufficiency is not the cause of the disease in humans. On the contrary, the *flatiron* mouse, a carrier of a *missense* heterozygous mutation, has impaired ferroportin membrane localization and suppressed iron export activity. In this model, mutant ferroportin has a dominant negative effect, preventing surface localization of wild-type ferroportin [27]. Due to the high serum ferritin level, low transferrin saturation, and iron loading of Kupffer cells, it is a mouse model for true ferroportin disease.

Clinical Features

The clinical presentation differs depending on the mutation type. In true ferroportin disease, transferrin saturation is normal or inappropriately low and iron is predominately stored in Kupffer cells. Serum ferritin is elevated and remains high despite phlebotomy: aggressive phlebotomy can provoke or aggravate anemia. Iron-related complications are absent or mild: even in the presence of severe iron burden, liver disease may be limited to sinusoidal fibrosis [1]. With increasing age, transferrin saturation and iron stores increase and iron is seen in hepatocytes as well as Kupffer cells.

Hemochromatosis due to 326 mutations mimics *HFE* hemochromatosis with high transferrin saturation, hepatocyte iron deposition, and liver cirrhosis. Unique clinical features were described by Ronald Sham in collaboration with the group of Ernest Beutler [28] in a large family along three generations in which some affected members, carriers of the Cys326Ser mutation, had liver disease, arthritis, elevated transferrin saturation, and hepatocyte iron storage even at a young age. A different amino-acid substitution at the same residue Cys326Tyr was described in Thailand [10] with a similar hemochromatosis phenotype. C326 is the residue essential for ferroportin binding to hepcidin in a short-sequence, highly conserved region, representing the hepcidin binding site [29]. This explains the unusual clinical manifestations suggestive of a juvenile dominant form.

Treatment

At present, patients with ferroportin mutations are treated as patients with classic hemochromatosis. However, it is unclear whether iron overload of Kupffer cells needs treatment. Some patients develop mild anemia and do not tolerate intensive phlebotomy. It is wise to apply less stringent protocols of phlebotomy to patients with true ferroportin disease, whereas patients with the hemochromatosis-like phenotype need the same treatment as classic hemochromatosis.

Digenic Inheritance

Rare cases presenting mutations in multiple genes have been published. The combination of mutations in *HFE* and *TFR2* genes produced a juvenile hemochromatosis-like phenotype in a single case, indicating that mutations in the two genes have an additive effect on iron loading [30]. To address the problem whether *HJV* or *HAMP* mutations may influence the phenotype of patients with adult-onset hemochromatosis, several groups have sequenced these genes in C282Y hemochromatosis or in patients without *HFE* mutations. Rarely, either the *HJV* or the *HAMP* mutation is associated with a more severe phenotype in these patients, but extensive family studies are lacking, and the effect is not seen in all cases.

To diagnose rare genetic forms of hemochromatosis is often an expensive and time-consuming procedure. However, to achieve the precise diagnosis of the different genetic forms may be important for family counseling and for appropriate prognostic and therapeutic approaches. Based on the present knowledge on digenic inheritance, screening for mutations in all hemochromatosis genes in search of multiple genetic lesions is not indicated.

References

1 Pietrangelo A: Hereditary hemochromatosis – a new look at an old disease. N Engl J Med 2004;350:2383–2397.
2 Camaschella C: Understanding iron homeostasis through genetic analysis of hemochromatosis and related disorders. Blood 2005;106:3710–3717.
3 De Gobbi M, Roetto A, Piperno A, Mariani R, Alberti F, Papanikolaou G, Politou M, Lockitch G, Girelli D, Fargion S, Cox TM, Gasparini P, Cazzola M, Camaschella C: Natural history of juvenile haemochromatosis. Br J Haematol 2002;117:973–979.
4 Roetto A, Papanikolaou G, Politou M, Alberti F, Girelli D, Christakis J, Loukopoulos D, Camaschella C: Mutant antimicrobial peptide hepcidin is associated with severe juvenile hemochromatosis. Nat Genet 2003;33:21–22.
5 Nemeth E, Tuttle MS, Powelson J, Vaughn MB, Donovan A, Ward DM, Ganz T, Kaplan J: Hepcidin regulates cellular iron efflux by binding to ferroportin and inducing its internalization. Science 2004;306:2090–2093.
6 Papanikolaou G, Samuels ME, Ludwig EH, MacDonald ML, Franchini PL, Dubé MP, Andres L, MacFarlane J, Sakellaropoulos N, Politou M, Nemeth E, Thompson J, Risler JK, Zaborowska C, Babakaiff R, Radomski CC, Pape TD, Davidas O, Christakis J, Brissot P, Lockitch G, Ganz T, Hayden MR, Goldberg YP: Mutations in HFE2 cause iron overload in chromosome 1q-linked juvenile hemochromatosis. Nat Genet 2004;36:77–82.
7 Lanzara C, Roetto A, Daraio F, Rivard S, Ficarella R, Simard H, Cox TM, Cazzola M, Piperno A, Gimenez-Roqueplo AP, Grammatico P, Volinia S, Gasparini P, Camaschella C: Spectrum of hemojuvelin gene mutations in 1q-linked juvenile hemochromatosis. Blood 2004;103:4317–4321.
8 Lee PL, Beutler E, Rao SV, Barton JC: Genetic abnormalities and juvenile hemochromatosis: mutations of the HJV gene encoding hemojuvelin. Blood 2004;103:4669–4671.
9 Koyama C, Hayashi H, Wakusawa S, Ueno T, Yano M, Katano Y, Goto H, Kidokoro R: Three patients with middle-age-onset hemochromatosis caused by novel mutations in the hemojuvelin gene. J Hepatol 2005;43:740–742.
10 Lok CY, Merryweather-Clarke AT, Viprakasit V, Chinthammitr Y, Srichairatanakool S, Limwongse C, Oleesky D, Robins AJ, Hudson J, Wai P, Premawardhena A, de Silva HJ, Dassanayake A, McKeown C, Jackson M, Gama R, Khan N, Newman W, Banait G, Chilton A, Wilson-Morkeh I, Weatherall DJ, Robson KJ: Iron overload in the Asian community. Blood 2009;114:20–25.

11 Babitt JL, Huang FW, Wrighting DM, Xia Y, Sidis Y, Samad TA, Campagna JA, Chung RT, Schneyer AL, Woolf CJ, Andrews NC, Lin HY: Bone morphogenetic protein signaling by hemojuvelin regulates hepcidin expression. Nat Genet 2006;38:531–539.
12 Niederkofler V, Salie R, Arber S: Hemojuvelin is essential for dietary iron sensing, and its mutation leads to severe iron overload. J Clin Invest 2005;115:2180–2186.
13 Meynard D, Kautz L, Darnaud V, Canonne-Hergaux F, Coppin H, Roth MP: Lack of the bone morphogenetic protein BMP6 induces massive iron overload. Nat Genet 2009;41:478–481.
14 Fabio G, Minonzio F, Delbini P, Bianchi A, Cappellini MD: Reversal of cardiac complications by deferiprone and deferoxamine combination therapy in a patient affected by a severe type of juvenile hemochromatosis (JH). Blood 2007;109:362–364.
15 Nick H, Allegrini PR, Fozard L, Junker U, Rojkjaer L, Salie R, Niederkofler V, O'Reilly T: Deferasirox reduces iron overload in a murine model of juvenile hemochromatosis. Exp Biol Med 2009;234:492–503.
16 Camaschella C, Roetto A: TFR2-related hereditary hemochromatosis; in: GeneReviews at GeneTests: Medical Genetics Information Resource (online database). Seattle, University of Washington, 1997–2005, available at http://www.genetests.org.
17 Camaschella C, Roetto A, Calì A, De Gobbi M, Garozzo G, Carella M, Majorano N, Totaro A, Gasparini P: The gene TFR2 is mutated in a new type of haemochromatosis mapping to 7q22. Nat Genet 2000;25:14–15.
18 Fleming RE, Ahmann JR, Migas MC, Waheed A, Koeffler HP, Kawabata H, Britton RS, Bacon BR, Sly WS: Targeted mutagenesis of the murine transferrin receptor-2 gene produces hemochromatosis. Proc Natl Acad Sci USA 2002;99:10653–10658.
19 Wallace DF, Summerville L, Subramaniam VN: Targeted disruption of the hepatic transferrin receptor 2 gene in mice leads to iron overload. Gastroenterology 2007;132:301–310.
20 Nemeth E, Roetto A, Garozzo G, Ganz T, Camaschella C: Hepcidin is decreased in TFR2 hemochromatosis. Blood 2005;105:1803–1806.

21 Girelli D, Bozzini C, Roetto A, Alberti F, Daraio F, Colombari R, Olivieri O, Corrocher R, Camaschella C: Clinical and pathologic findings in hemochromatosis type 3 due to a novel mutation in transferrin receptor 2 gene. Gastroenterology 2002;122:1295–1302.
22 Njajou OT, Vaessen N, Joosse M, Berghuis B, van Dongen JW, Breuning MH, Snijders PJ, Rutten WP, Sandkuijl LA, Oostra BA, van Duijn CM, Heutink P: A mutation in SLC11A3 is associated with autosomal dominant hemochromatosis. Nat Genet 2001;28:213–214.
23 Montosi G, Donovan A, Totaro A, Garuti C, Pignatti E, Cassanelli S, Trenor CC, Gasparini P, Andrews NC, Pietrangelo A: Autosomal-dominant hemochromatosis is associated with a mutation in the ferroportin (SLC11A3) gene. J Clin Invest 2001;108:619–623.
24 Wallace DF, Subramaniam VN: Non-HFE haemochromatosis. World J Gastroenterol 2007;13:4690–4698.
25 Fernandes A, Preza GC, Phung Y, De Domenico I, Kaplan J, Ganz T, Nemeth E: The molecular basis of hepcidin-resistant hereditary hemochromatosis. Blood 2009;114:437–443.
26 De Domenico I, Ward DM, Musci G, Kaplan J: Iron overload due to mutations in ferroportin. Haematologica 2006;91:92–95.
27 Zohn IE, De Domenico I, Pollock A, Ward DM, Goodman JF, Liang X, Sanchez AJ, Niswander L, Kaplan J: The flatiron mutation in mouse ferroportin acts as a dominant negative to cause ferroportin disease. Blood 2007;109:4174–4180.
28 Sham RL, Phatak PD, West C, Lee P, Andrews C, Beutler E: Autosomal dominant hereditary hemochromatosis associated with a novel ferroportin mutation and unique clinical features. Blood Cells Mol Dis 2005;34:157–161.
29 De Domenico I, Nemeth E, Nelson JM, Phillips JD, Ajioka RS, Kay MS, Kushner JP, Ganz T, Ward DM, Kaplan J: The hepcidin-binding site on ferroportin is evolutionarily conserved. Cell Metab 2008;8:146–156.
30 Pietrangelo A, Caleffi A, Henrion J, Ferrara F, Corradini E, Kulaksiz H, Stremmel W, Andreone P, Garuti C: Juvenile hemochromatosis associated with pathogenic mutations of adult hemochromatosis genes. Gastroenterology 2005;128:470–479.

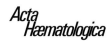

Acta Haematol 2009;122:146–154
DOI: 10.1159/000243799

Published online: November 10, 2009

Role of T2* Magnetic Resonance in Monitoring Iron Chelation Therapy

John-Paul Carpenter   Dudley J. Pennell

Cardiovascular Magnetic Resonance Unit, Royal Brompton Hospital, London, UK

Key Words

Cardiac complications · Chelation · Magnetic resonance imaging · Monitoring of thalassaemia patients · Myocardial siderosis · T2* · Thalassaemia

Abstract

The monitoring of chelation therapy is a very important part of the management of transfusion-dependent patients. Classical methods of monitoring iron loading are either unreliable or unable to detect important myocardial siderosis which can predispose to the development of cardiac complications such as heart failure. The development of the T2* technique using cardiovascular magnetic resonance has allowed clinicians to have a reliable method for measuring cardiac iron to guide chelation therapy. T2* can identify early those patients who are at risk of developing cardiac complications, enabling personalised, tailored therapy to avoid potential problems.   Copyright © 2009 S. Karger AG, Basel

Introduction

Worldwide, there are many hundreds of thousands of patients born each year with severe haemoglobinopathies. The majority of these births are sickle cell disease, but of at least 40,000 born with β-thalassaemia major (TM), an estimated 25,000 require regular transfusions to survive. The ultimate aim of monitoring chelation therapy is to ensure that iron loading resulting from the transfusions is kept to a minimum in order to prevent tissue damage, organ dysfunction and adverse outcomes. Each unit of transfused blood contains approximately 250 mg of elemental iron and with no physiological excretory mechanism, the human body is unable to get rid of the excess iron. This iron accumulates in organs and tissues, the most serious complication being death from cardiac failure due to myocardial siderosis. In the era before chelation therapy, the natural history of severe iron overload was very evident. Transfusion-dependent patients developed cardiac enlargement by the age of 10 followed by heart block, pericarditis, atrial arrhythmias and heart failure. The mean age at onset of cardiac failure was 16 years, with more than half of the affected patients dying within a year of heart failure becoming apparent. In general, the prognosis was extremely poor and most died before the age of 20. The introduction of deferoxamine in the late 1970s changed all this with a dramatically improved prognosis for survival free from cardiac disease. Even patients who had developed heart failure were able to survive longer, with 48% still alive 5 years after disease onset. However, until recently, despite routine chelation therapy, overall outcomes were still poor

Prof. Dudley J. Pennell
Cardiovascular Magnetic Resonance Unit, Royal Brompton Hospital
Sydney Street
London, SW3 6NP (UK)
Tel. +44 207 351 8810, Fax +44 207 351 8816, E-Mail d.pennell@imperial.ac.uk

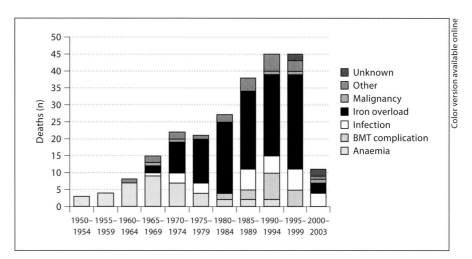

Fig. 1. Numbers of deceased TM patients in the UK. There has been a 71% reduction in the annualised death rate from cardiovascular causes due to iron overload since 2000. The number of deaths in the 2000–2003 interval represents the number of deaths in a 4-year period but in all other groups, the number of deaths is over 5 years (reproduced with permission [2]). BMT = Bone marrow transplantation.

with up to 50% of the patients dying by the age of 35 years and 71% as a direct result of cardiac siderosis [1]. Recent advances in chelation therapy, improvements in patient management and the widespread implementation of cardiac T2* measurement have had a major impact on improving survival, and in the UK since the year 2000, there has been a 71% reduction in the death rate attributable to cardiovascular deaths from cardiac iron overload (fig. 1) [2].

Techniques for Assessing Tissue Iron

The onset of detectable ventricular impairment is a late manifestation of severe cardiac iron loading and, therefore, early detection of cardiac siderosis is essential. Traditional monitoring techniques used for the assessment of cardiac iron loading and ventricular function all have significant shortcomings. Although echocardiography is a widely available non-invasive technique which provides good measurement of left-ventricular (LV) function, changes in diastolic parameters or ejection fraction (EF) do not become apparent until there has been a prolonged period of severe cardiac iron loading. Tissue Doppler and strain imaging does detect some abnormal parameters even in young, asymptomatic and well-chelated patients, but it is not clear how this relates to clinical outcomes. Serum ferritin is still regularly measured in routine clinical practice but can be misleading. Although serial measurements may provide an overall idea of iron loading in a particular patient, it only represents 1% of the total body iron and is an imprecise assessment of total iron storage. Among other factors, it is an acute-phase

protein which makes it an unreliable marker in the context of acute illness or infection. Direct measurement of liver iron concentration (LIC) can give a good appreciation of the liver iron levels, but liver biopsy is an invasive procedure with non-negligible risks. LIC levels are also affected by fibrosis and the degree of heterogeneity of iron loading within the liver. Unfortunately, neither serum ferritin nor LIC bears any useful clinical relationship to myocardial iron loading [3]. Techniques which rely on biomagnetic susceptometry, such as iron measurement by superconducting quantum interference device, can be useful for guiding chelation therapy regimens based on liver iron but have a very limited availability worldwide and cannot be used to measure iron in the heart. Endomyocardial biopsy measures the iron concentration of myocardial biopsy samples from the right-ventricular endocardial surface of the interventricular septum but is an invasive procedure (once again with associated risks) which may be affected by the heterogeneity of iron loading in the septum and limited access to experienced operators. Therefore, in the late 1990s, the development of non-invasive measurement of cardiac iron concentration became the 'Holy Grail' of the monitoring of chelation therapy.

Pathophysiology of Iron Loading

Iron is essential for normal cellular function and at normal physiological levels, plasma iron is bound to transferrin, preventing any catalytic activity and free radical formation. Under conditions of iron overload, the transferrin becomes saturated and iron appears in the plasma in its free form (non-transferrin-bound iron). The iron enters cells and is stored as soluble ferritin or insoluble haemosiderin particles but once this storage capacity is exceeded, excess iron within myocytes enters a labile iron pool which can have a catalytic role in the initiation of free radical reactions and a detrimental effect on cardiac function. There is increased lysosomal fragility and iron-induced peroxidative damage to membrane proteins and lipids. The non-transferrin-bound iron also causes cellular damage by effects on the mitochondrial respiratory chain and by impaired Na-K-ATPase activity. Iron chelators have been shown to reverse this process. Ex vivo studies of deferoxamine and deferiprone in cultured myocytes have demonstrated that these agents can bind the labile iron and remove it from the cells, reversing the lipid peroxidation, the impairment in the Na-K-ATPase and the iron-induced abnormalities of cardiac contractile function [4]. Whilst magnetic resonance (MR) does not detect soluble free iron, the particulate iron in the form of haemosiderin in the heart prompted the idea that this could be exploited to measure iron concentrations.

Measurement of Cardiac Iron Concentration Using Cardiovascular MR

The concept which underlies the technique is simple. Cardiovascular MR (CMR) uses the combination of a strong magnetic field and radiofrequency pulses to generate images. Protons (hydrogen nuclei) align along the axis of the main magnetic field within the scanner and can be deflected by a radiofrequency pulse. Following such a pulse, their transverse magnetisation decays exponentially back towards zero. The rate of decay of transverse magnetisation and the recovery of the original magnetisation is determined by the relaxation parameters T1 (longitudinal relaxation) and T2 (transverse relaxation). T2* is a form of T2 with higher sensitivity to field changes caused by iron. Tissue iron can be measured indirectly from the effect of particulate iron within myocytes on relaxation times of hydrogen nuclei. The presence of iron causes a local disruption of the magnetic field, thereby shortening the relaxation times and these quantifiable effects can be calibrated for absolute iron concentration.

There are a number of techniques which have been used to try and assess myocardial iron concentration using CMR. Signal intensity ratios compare the signal of the myocardium to that of another reference tissue, such as skeletal muscle, assuming that there is little or no iron loading within this tissue. This method was initially developed for measurement of liver iron, but subsequent attempts have been made to calibrate the measurement of myocardial/muscle signal intensity ratios for iron concentration [5]. This method has not proven reliable as it makes a number of assumptions including the calculation of cardiac iron concentration from a modified calibration curve derived from the liver. As well as this, there can be a significant variation in results obtained with only minor changes in imaging parameters.

T2 techniques are useful for measuring liver iron as the T2 can be directly measured and does not require a reference tissue for comparison [6]. However, the application of T2 relaxivity to the heart is more difficult due to problems associated with hardware constraints, blood flow, cardiac motion and noise, which affect the accuracy and reproducibility of the measurement. T2 has been shown to correlate with myocardial iron concentration in animals and has also been compared with endomyocardial biopsy samples in humans [7, 8]. Recent improvements in scanner technology have allowed the development of T2 sequences which can be applied to cardiac scanning, but further work is required before this becomes a useful clinical tool [9].

T2* is quicker and easier to measure in the heart than T2, is more sensitive to iron and less sensitive to cardiac motion. In a single breath-hold, a series of images of the heart are acquired at different echo times following a radiofrequency pulse, each image getting progressively darker as the signal fades (fig. 2) [10]. Intracellular iron causes signal intensity to decay away faster and the higher the iron concentration within the myocyte, the faster the signal decay. If signal intensity is plotted against the echo time of each image, an exponential decay curve is seen. The curve equation is of the form $y = ke^{-(TE/T2^*)}$, where k is a constant and TE is the echo time. The decay constant T2* (measured in ms) can be derived from this equation and can be considered as the time taken for 63% of the signal to have been lost (fig. 3).

When the T2* technique was first developed, not only were multiple breath-holds required but it was noted that there were significant imaging artefacts from deoxygenated blood in the cardiac veins and fat in the atrioventricular groove. This is because T2* is influenced by small-scale inhomogeneities which occur at tissue interfaces such as the liver/myocardial border at the LV inferior wall and the lung/myocardial border at the LV lateral wall. As a result, a mid-ventricular short-axis slice was chosen with a region of interest in the septum to give a uniform myocardial segment free of artefact for the

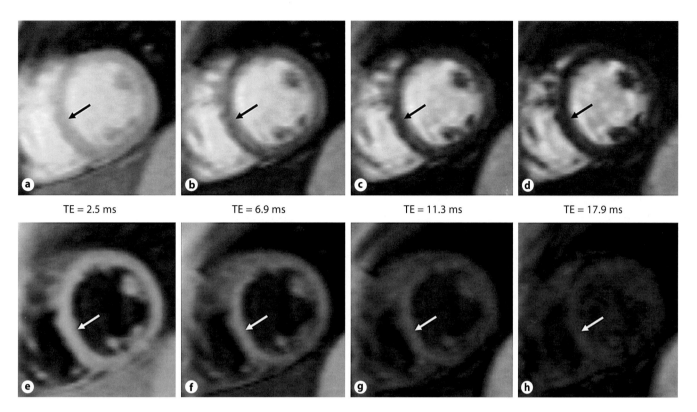

Fig. 2. T2* images of the heart. This set of images shows both bright-blood (**a–d**) and dark-blood (**e–h**) T2* acquisitions of a mid-ventricular short-axis slice through the heart. Myocardial signal intensity (arrows) becomes darker with increasing echo time (TE).

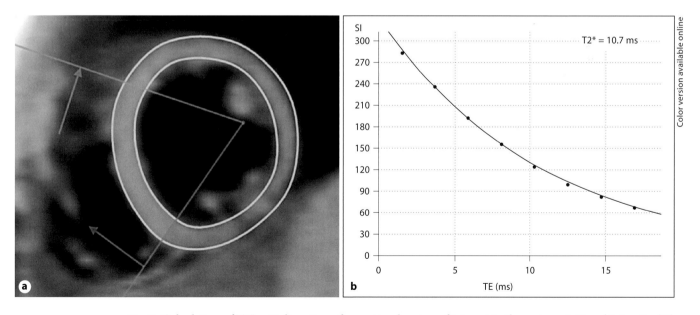

Fig. 3. Calculation of T2*. **a** Delineation of an optimal region of interest in the septum. **b** Signal intensity (SI) on the vertical axis plotted against echo time (TE). The calculated T2* value is 10.7 ms, reflecting moderate myocardial iron loading.

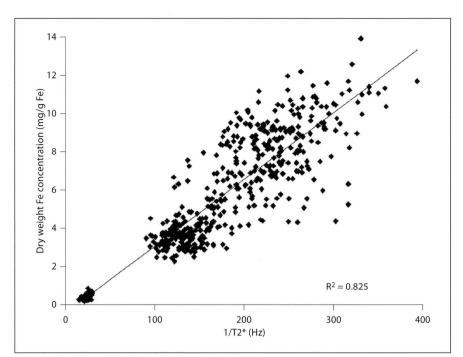

Fig. 4. Calibration of cardiac T2* for absolute iron concentration. Preliminary data from a series of post-mortem hearts in which T2* (measured in multiple regions of interest) was compared with absolute iron concentration measured by atomic emission spectrometry. Iron concentration on the vertical axis is plotted against the reciprocal of T2* (reproduced with permission [14]).

measurement of T2* decay. This technique gives a single value for cardiac T2*, which is representative of the iron loading throughout the heart [3, 11]. The normal range for T2* (derived from a group of normal individuals with no history of transfusion or cardiac disease) is 52 ± 16 ms, with a median normal value of 40 ms. The lower limit of the normal range is 20 ms. Myocardial infarction, ischaemia and haemorrhage can cause T2* shortening, but there are no clinical reports other than in patients with iron loading of T2* being <20 ms [3].

Other groups have suggested that a whole-heart T2* map could be generated from multiple slices, measuring T2* in all segments of the heart with a correction algorithm from scans of normal volunteers to try and remove any artefact [12]. Using this method, significant regional heterogeneity in T2* values has been reported but there are no clinical data relating these findings to outcomes, and the measurement from a single large region of interest in the septum is highly representative of mean cardiac iron.

T2* Measurement of Cardiac Iron

Cardiac T2* bears a direct relationship to the myocardial iron concentration. This has been demonstrated in an animal model of iron loading which mimics the

iron overload seen in transfusion-dependent patients. In the gerbil, a linear correlation was found between absolute iron concentration and 1/T2*, and a calibration for T2* versus iron concentration was derived for both heart and liver. Even without an absolute calibration for human heart tissue, the findings supported the use of CMR to evaluate iron loading in humans [7]. Subsequently, a single post-mortem heart from a patient with TM who died of overwhelming biliary sepsis was scanned and T2* values were compared to absolute iron concentrations in multiple regions of the myocardium. 1/T2* rose linearly with iron concentration, but the limited range of iron values precluded a wide-ranging absolute calibration [13]. Preliminary data regarding the calibration of T2* versus absolute iron concentrations measured by atomic emission spectroscopy in post-mortem hearts from TM patients with a range of iron loading have been reported, and it is clear that there is a relationship between 1/T2* in the human heart and iron concentration (fig. 4) [14].

Relationship between T2* and Ventricular Function

The measurement of LV and right ventricular volumes and function with CMR is highly reproducible and is now considered to be the 'gold standard' for ventricular assessment. As a result, this provides an important part of the assessment and longitudinal follow-up for patients at risk of myocardial iron overload, but patients with chronic anemia have different normal ranges for LV parameters than non-transfused, non-anemic subjects. Those with TM who have no evidence of cardiac iron loading have a higher indexed end-diastolic volume, LV stroke volume and LVEF with a lower end-diastolic volume [15]. This has an important impact on the monitoring of chelation therapy as a low EF in TM may signify the onset of LV impairment due to myocardial siderosis even though it is still within the accepted range for normal individuals. When T2* is >20 ms, the majority of TM patients have LVEF within the normal range. As T2* falls below 20 ms, LVEF also falls with the most marked decline seen in those with T2* <10 ms [3]. The same effect is seen with right ventricular function and LV diastolic parameters. The great majority of patients who develop symptoms and clinical evidence of cardiac failure have T2* values <10 ms [16].

Reproducibility of T2* Measurements

Despite the fact that T2* is easy and quick to acquire, it is a very robust, reliable technique. Using dedicated software (ThalassaemiaTools, a plug-in for CMRtools; Cardiovascular Imaging Solutions, London, UK), the interobserver reproducibility is good with a coefficient of variation of 6.4% for the heart and 4.5% for the liver [3]. The interstudy reproducibility has also been proven by performing two separate CMR scans, either within the same week for the multiple breath-hold technique or on the same day for the single breath-hold technique (with a mean interval of 20 min between scans). For the multiple breath-hold technique, the coefficient of variation was 3.3% for the liver and 5.0% for the heart [3]. For the multi-echo single breath-hold technique, the coefficient of variation between scans was 2.3% for patients with T2* <20 ms and 5.8% for all patients [10]. The worldwide agreement between sites and the validity of the technique for different vendor platforms has been studied using scanners from all of the major CMR manufacturers and comparing the results to a reference site in London. Patients who had undergone a local T2* scan were flown from sites in the USA and Europe to London for a reference scan. The overall reproducibility for heart and liver T2* was 5.0 and 7.1%, with mean absolute differences in T2* of 1.3 and 0.45 ms, respectively [17].

T2* and Liver Iron

Liver T2* can be measured using a technique similar to that for the heart, but with shorter echo times, because the higher iron concentration within the liver can lead to very short T2* values. A multi-echo single breath-hold scan generates a set of images through a transverse slice of the liver. A region of interest (chosen in a homogeneous area of liver tissue to avoid artefact from blood vessels) is used to derive a similar decay curve from which T2* can be calculated. When compared to LIC from non-fibrotic liver biopsy samples, there was a strong linear relationship between LIC and T2* when log transformed (R = 0.93, p < 0.0001). As a result of this work, a calibration was derived for T2* versus LIC [3]. Once again, this has been confirmed in animal models [7]. Updated, more modern scanner hardware with stronger and faster gradients has allowed the echo times to be shortened and this is likely to allow more accurate measurement of T2*, especially at higher levels of liver iron loading.

Relationship between Myocardial T2*, Serum Ferritin and Liver Iron

When compared to cardiac T2*, serum ferritin values show no clinically useful relationship. While there is a trend towards higher ferritin levels at lower myocardial T2* values, indicating higher degrees of iron loading, the correlation is too weak to have any value [3, 11]. A similar problem has been noted with respect to liver iron loading. When liver T2* and cardiac T2* values are compared, there is wide discrepancy with some patients having very low liver T2* (signifying high liver iron) and high cardiac T2* (no cardiac iron loading). The converse may also be true in that some patients can have almost no iron loading in the liver but severe cardiac iron overload (as measured by T2*) [3]. This only became apparent with the development of the cardiac T2* technique and may explain why patients with good total body iron values (low ferritin and low LIC) can still develop cardiac failure [18]. These findings reinforce that neither LIC nor ferritin can be used as a surrogate measurement of cardiac iron.

Trials of Chelation Therapy Involving T2*

An initial prospective study of TM patients who all presented with overt symptoms of heart failure assessed the relationship of T2* to ventricular function, heart failure and intensive chelation therapy [19]. All 7 patients had severe myocardial iron loading at baseline with a mean cardiac T2* value of 5.1 ± 1.9 ms and underwent intensive chelation therapy with intravenous deferoxamine via indwelling central venous catheter (mean dosage 42–51 mg/kg/day). One patient died shortly after the initial scan but in those who survived, there was a progressive and significant improvement in LV ejection fraction over the course of 1 year (from 52 to 63%; p = 0.03) associated with an improvement in T2* (to 8.1 ± 2.8 ms; p = 0.003) and an improvement in symptoms according to the New York Heart Association class. Although the improvement in cardiac T2* was significant, the rate of improvement was significantly slower ($5.0 \pm 3.3\%$ per month) in comparison to the improvement in T2* seen in the liver ($39 \pm 23\%$ per month; p = 0.02).

A second prospective study involving 22 patients with severe cardiac iron loading (T2* <8 ms) and impaired LV function confirmed the reversible nature of the cardiomyopathy [20]. Rather than intravenous chelation therapy, all patients were prescribed a combination of subcutaneous deferoxamine (38 ± 10.2 mg/kg for 5.3 days/week) and oral deferiprone (73.9 ± 4.0 mg/kg/day) for 1 year. Myocardial T2* improved from 5.7 to 7.9 ms (p = 0.010), with an associated improvement in LVEF from 51.2 to 65.6% (p < 0.001). Liver iron loading also improved, with liver T2* increasing from 3.7 to 10.8 ms (p = 0.006). Once again, in this cohort with severe iron loading, liver T2* and LVEF appeared to improve much more rapidly than cardiac T2*.

These two studies have not only confirmed that the cardiac failure secondary to siderotic cardiomyopathy is reversible, but have shown that T2* improves in parallel with the improvement in LVEF, LV volumes and symptoms. The improvement in myocardial T2* seems to lag behind the improvement in EF. This is thought to be the result of a two-stage process as the chelation agents rapidly remove the labile iron pool in the myocytes first (leading to an improvement in ventricular volumes and EF) with a slower removal of the stored myocardial iron, limited by the rate of removal of haemosiderin. Within the liver, there is a facilitated uptake and excretion pathway for deferoxamine, and the metabolism and turnover of hepatic ferritin is much faster. The fact that cardiac iron improves slowly has important implications for the treatment of patients with heart failure. Regardless of the improvement in LVEF, it is important to persevere with intensive chelation treatment until T2* has improved.

There have been several randomised controlled trials (some of which are still in progress) looking at the effects of different iron chelators on myocardial iron loading using change in myocardial siderosis (cardiac T2*) as their primary end-point. The first of these was the LA16 trial which randomised 61 patients (who had been previously maintained on subcutaneous deferoxamine) to either switch to oral deferiprone monotherapy or remain on subcutaneous deferoxamine for the duration of 1 year [21]. The inclusion criteria required patients to have an abnormal, but not severe level of myocardial iron loading (T2* between 8 and 20 ms) with LVEF >56% (the lower limit of the normal range for healthy, non-anaemic subjects). At the end of the trial, there was a reduction in myocardial siderosis in both groups, however the improvement in myocardial T2* was significantly greater for deferiprone than deferoxamine (27 vs. 13%; p = 0.023). LVEF also increased significantly more in the deferiprone-treated group (3.1 vs. 0.3% absolute units; p = 0.003). A subsequent double-blind, placebo controlled trial looking to assess the effects of combination therapy randomised patients to either subcutaneous deferoxamine and oral deferiprone or deferoxamine and placebo [22]. In the combined treatment group taking the active drug, myocardial T2* improved significantly from a baseline of 11.7 to 14.7 ms at 6 months and 17.7 ms at 12 months (p = 0.001). In the group taking only deferoxamine, myocardial T2* increased from a baseline of 12.4–14.5 ms at 6 months to 15.7 ms at 12 months (p = 0.001). When the two groups were compared, there was a significantly greater increase in cardiac T2* in the combined treatment group (p = 0.02). Liver T2* values improved significantly in both groups, but there was a far greater improvement in the combination group (p < 0.001). LVEF also improved to a greater degree in the combination group from 65.8% at baseline to 68.4% at 12 months in comparison to the deferoxamine group where LVEF was unchanged (64.7 vs. 65.3%) at 12 months (p = 0.05).

Large multicentre trials involving the new oral chelator deferasirox are still ongoing (the Novartis 2206 trial is due to report in December 2011). For the cardiac substudies, the primary end-point has been defined as the change in T2* from baseline to 1 year with secondary end-points being improvement in LV volumes and LVEF. Non-randomised results with deferasirox show it removes cardiac iron, but with no significant change in EF at 12 months. EF changes may occur with deferasirox when cardiac iron levels are near normal [23].

Prognostic Value of T2*

It has been demonstrated that LVEF decreases with worsening myocardial T2* and that patients with a very low T2* are at risk of symptomatic heart failure and ventricular arrhythmias (the majority of patients who present with heart failure due to siderotic cardiomyopathy having a T2* <10 ms) [11, 16]. The trials mentioned above have elucidated that intensive chelation therapy improves myocardial T2* and results in amelioration of LVEF. However, it has not yet been proven that this translates into direct clinical benefit. A preliminary report of a large, prospective, observational study involving 652 patients has suggested that the lowest values of myocardial T2* (<10 ms) predict a high risk of the development of cardiac failure [24]. Analysis of T2* revealed an increasing risk of developing heart failure with progressively lower T2* values. In comparison to patients with T2* >20 ms, there was a significantly higher risk of developing heart failure with T2* <10 ms (p < 0.001), but the greatest risk of heart failure was in those patients with T2* <6 ms (p < 0.001). As a result, a simple traffic-light guide of cardiac risk ranges can be used: a T2* value >20 ms indicates a low risk, 10–20 ms an intermediate risk and <10 ms a high risk of cardiovascular events.

Conclusions

The development of the T2* technique is a prime example of translational research. The basic physical principles have been developed into a validated clinical application which has been proven in research trials. We now know that T2* measures cardiac iron, is highly reproducible and has the potential to determine prognosis for individual patients. It can be used to monitor chelation, allowing individually tailored chelation therapy to improve outcomes and prevent cardiovascular complications.

Disclosures

Prof. Dudley J. Pennell
Novartis: Consultancy, speakers honoraria, principal investigator of two Novartis studies (2409 and 2206), Research Funding; *Siemens:* Consultancy, Research Funding; *Cardiovascular Imaging Solutions:* Equity Ownership; *ApoPharma:* Consultancy, Speaker's honoraria.

Dr. John-Paul Carpenter
Swedish Orphan: Honoraria.

References

1 Modell B, Khan M, Darlison M: Survival in beta thalassaemia major in the UK: data from the UK Thalassaemia Register. Lancet 2000;355:2051–2052.

2 Modell B, Khan M, Darlison M, Westwood MA, Ingram D, Pennell DJ: Improved survival of thalassaemia major in the UK and relation to T2* cardiovascular magnetic resonance. J Cardiovasc Magn Reson 2008;10:42.

3 Anderson LJ, Holden S, Davis B, Prescott E, Charrier CC, Bunce NH, Firmin DN, Wonke B, Porter J, Walker JM, Pennell DJ: Cardiovascular T2-star (T2*) magnetic resonance for the early diagnosis of myocardial iron overload. Eur Heart J 2001;22:2171–2179.

4 Link G, Pinson A, Hershko C: Ability of the orally effective iron chelators dimethyl- and diethyl-hydroxypyrid-4-one and of deferoxamine to restore sarcolemmal thiolic enzyme activity in iron-loaded heart cells. Blood 1994;83:2692–2697.

5 Jensen PD, Jensen FT, Christensen T, Heickendorff L, Jensen LG, Ellegaard J: Indirect evidence for the potential ability of magnetic resonance imaging to evaluate the myocardial iron content in patients with transfu-

sional iron overload. MAGMA 2001;12:153–166.

6 St Pierre TG, Clark PR, Chua-Anusorn W: Single spin-echo proton transverse relaxometry of iron-loaded liver. NMR Biomed 2004;17:446–458.

7 Wood JC, Otto-Duessel M, Aguilar M, Nick H, Nelson MD, Coates TD, Pollack H, Moats R: Cardiac iron determines cardiac T2*, T2, and T1 in the gerbil model of iron cardiomyopathy. Circulation 2005;112:535–543.

8 Mavrogeni SI, Markussis V, Kaklamanis L, Tsiapras D, Paraskevaidis I, Karavolias G, Karagiorga M, Douskou M, Cokkinos DV, Kremastinos DT: A comparison of magnetic resonance imaging and cardiac biopsy in the evaluation of heart iron overload in patients with beta-thalassemia major. Eur J Haematol 2005;75:241–247.

9 He T, Gatehouse PD, Anderson LJ, Tanner M, Keegan J, Pennell DJ, Firmin DN: Development of a novel optimized breathhold technique for myocardial T2 measurement in thalassemia. J Magn Reson Imaging 2006;24:580–585.

10 Westwood M, Anderson LJ, Firmin DN, Gatehouse PD, Charrier CC, Wonke B, Pen-

nell DJ: A single breath-hold multiecho T2* cardiovascular magnetic resonance technique for diagnosis of myocardial iron overload. J Magn Reson Imaging 2003;18:33–39.

11 Wood JC, Tyszka JM, Carson S, Nelson MD, Coates TD: Myocardial iron loading in transfusion-dependent thalassemia and sickle cell disease. Blood 2004;103:1934–1936.

12 Ramazzotti A, Pepe A, Positano V, Scattini B, Santarelli MF, Landini L, De Marchi D, Keilberg P, Derchi G, Formisano F, Pili M, Lai ME, Forni G, Filosa A, Prossomariti L, Capra M, Pitrolo L, Borgna-Pignatti C, Cianciulli P, Maggio A, Lombardi M: Standardized T2* map of a normal human heart to correct T2* segmental artifacts. Myocardial iron overload and fibrosis in thalassemia intermedia versus thalassemia major patients and electrocardiogram changes in thalassemia major patients. Hemoglobin 2008;32:97–107.

13 Ghugre NR, Enriquez CM, Gonzalez I, Nelson MD Jr, Coates TD, Wood JC: MRI detects myocardial iron in the human heart. Magn Reson Med 2006;56:681–686.

14 Carpenter JP, He T, Kirk P, Anderson LJ, Porter JB, Wood JC, Galanello R, Forni G, Catani G, Fucharoen S, Fleming A, House M, Black G, Firmin DN, St Pierre TG, Pennell DJ: Calibration of myocardial iron concentration against T2-star cardiovascular magnetic resonance. J Cardiovasc Magn Reson 2009;11(suppl 1):P224.

15 Westwood MA, Anderson LJ, Maceira AM, Shah FT, Prescott E, Porter JB, Wonke B, Walker JM, Pennell DJ: Normalized left ventricular volumes and function in thalassemia major patients with normal myocardial iron. J Magn Reson Imaging 2007;25:1147–1151.

16 Tanner MA, Porter JB, Westwood MA, Nair SV, Anderson LJ, Walker JM, Pennell DJ: Myocardial T2* in patients with cardiac failure secondary to iron overload (abstract). Blood 2005;106:3838.

17 Tanner MA, He T, Westwood MA, Firmin DN, Pennell DJ, Thalassemia International Federation Heart T2* Investigators: Multicenter validation of the transferability of the magnetic resonance T2* technique for the quantification of tissue iron. Haematologica 2006;91:1388–1391.

18 Anderson LJ, Westwood MA, Prescott E, Walker JM, Pennell DJ, Wonke B: Development of thalassaemic iron overload cardiomyopathy despite low liver iron levels and meticulous compliance to desferrioxamine. Acta Haematol 2006;115:106–108.

19 Anderson LJ, Westwood MA, Holden S, Davis B, Prescott E, Wonke B, Porter JB, Walker JM, Pennell DJ: Myocardial iron clearance during reversal of siderotic cardiomyopathy with intravenous desferrioxamine: a prospective study using T2* cardiovascular magnetic resonance. Br J Haematol 2004; 127:348–355.

20 Tanner MA, Galanello R, Dessi C, Smith GC, Westwood MA, Agus A, Pibiri M, Nair SV, Walker JM, Pennell DJ: Combined chelation therapy in thalassemia major for the treatment of severe myocardial siderosis with left ventricular dysfunction. J Cardiovasc Magn Reson 2008;10:12.

21 Pennell DJ, Berdoukas V, Karagiorga M, Ladis V, Piga A, Aessopos A, Gotsis S, Tanner MA, Smith GC, Westwood MA, Wonke B, Galanello R: Randomized controlled trial of the effect of deferiprone or deferoxamine on myocardial iron and function in beta-thalassemia major. Blood 2006;107:3738–3744.

22 Tanner MA, Galanello R, Dessi C, Smith GC, Westwood MA, Agus A, Roughton M, Assomull R, Nair SV, Walker JM, Pennell DJ: A randomized, placebo-controlled, double-blind trial of the effect of combined therapy with deferoxamine and deferiprone on myocardial iron in thalassemia major using cardiovascular magnetic resonance. Circulation 2007;115:1876–1884.

23 Pennell DJ, Porter J, Cappellini MD, Chi-Kong L, Aydinok Y, Lee CL, Kattamis A, Smith GC, Habr D, Domokos G, Hmissi A, Taher A: Efficacy and safety of deferasirox (Exjade) in reducing cardiac iron in patients with beta-thalassemia major: results from the cardiac substudy of the EPIC trial (abstract). Blood 2008;112:3873.

24 Kirk P, Roughton M, Porter JB, Walker JM, Tanner MA, Patel J, Wu D, Taylor J, Westwood MA, Anderson LJ, Pennel DJ: Cardiac T2* magnetic resonance for prediction of cardiac complications in thalassemia major (abstract). J Cardiovasc Magn Reson 2009; 11(suppl 1):O2.

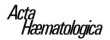

Acta Haematol 2009;122:155–164
DOI: 10.1159/000243800

Published online: November 10, 2009

Deferiprone Chelation Therapy for Thalassemia Major

R. Galanello   S. Campus

Dipartimento di Scienze Biomediche e Biotecnologie, Ospedale Regionale Microcitemie,
Azienda Sanitaria Locale 8, Università di Cagliari, Cagliari, Italia

Key Words
Chelation · Combination therapy · Deferiprone ·
Gastrointestinal symptoms · Myocardial siderosis ·
Thalassemia major

Abstract
Iron overload is one of the major causes of morbidity in patients with thalassemia major. Deferiprone (DFP), an orally active iron chelator, emerged from an extensive search for new drugs to treat iron overload. Comparative studies have shown that at comparable doses the efficacy of DFP in removing body iron is similar to that of desferoxamine (DFO). In retrospective and prospective studies, DFP monotherapy was significantly more effective than DFO in the treatment of myocardial siderosis in thalassemia major. DFP can be used in combination with DFO in the management of severe iron overload. This chelation regimen is tolerable and attractive for patients unable to comply with standard DFO infusions or with inadequate response to DFP monotherapy. DFP has a well-known long-term safety profile. Agranulocytosis is the most serious side effect associated with its use, occurring in about 1% of the patients. More common but less serious side effects are gastrointestinal symptoms, arthralgia, zinc deficiency, and fluctuating transaminase levels.

Copyright © 2009 S. Karger AG, Basel

Introduction

Deferiprone (1,2-dimethyl-3-hydroxypyrid-4-one, also known as L1, DFP, CP20, and Ferriprox) is a 'new' iron chelator first used in humans in 1987 [1].

It belongs to the hydroxypyridone class of iron chelators and was designed in 1984 at the University of Essex in London as a potentially useful compound for the management of clinical iron overload [2]. They were searching for a molecule that could be taken orally, bind iron in the condition of iron overload, e.g. thalassemia, and excrete it from the body. The compound was first screened in cells lines; subsequently, it was tested in an animal model of iron overload, proving that it was absorbed by the gastrointestinal (GI) apparatus and caused excretion of excess iron [3].

Iron is indispensable for the survival of virtually all life forms, being involved in many essential metabolic pathways. However, it is noteworthy that the human body has no active mechanism for iron excretion [4]. Consequently, in conditions of primary (hereditary hemochromatosis) or secondary (e.g. thalassemia major) iron overload, accumulation of this potentially toxic element results in massive buildup of iron. Iron stored in reticuloendothelial and parenchymal cells rapidly reaches and exceeds the levels that can be controlled by normal homeostatic mechanisms. Excess iron in the

Renzo Galanello
Ospedale Regionale Microcitemie
Via Jenner s/n
IT–09121 Cagliari (Italy)
Tel. +39 070 609 5508, Fax +39 070 609 5509, E-Mail renzo.galanello@mcweb.unica.it

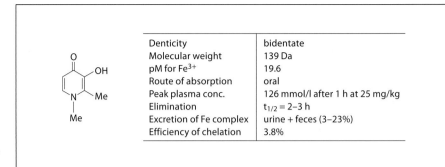

Fig. 1. Structure and pharmacologic properties of DFP.

Denticity	bidentate
Molecular weight	139 Da
pM for Fe^{3+}	19.6
Route of absorption	oral
Peak plasma conc.	126 mmol/l after 1 h at 25 mg/kg
Elimination	$t_{1/2}$ = 2–3 h
Excretion of Fe complex	urine + feces (3–23%)
Efficiency of chelation	3.8%

body saturates the associated iron-binding proteins transferrin and ferritin, leading to the appearance of the highly reactive free forms of iron: non-transferrin-bound iron in the plasma and labile cellular iron in the cells [5, 6]. Free iron is toxic to cells acting as a catalyst in the formation of free radicals from reactive oxygen species via the Fenton reaction. Within the cells, iron toxicity occurs when pools of intracellular labile iron accumulate and mediate tissue damage via the formation of harmful reactive oxygen species. Peroxidation of intracellular organelles (lysosomes and mitochondria) and membrane components by reactive oxygen species is the major cause of iron-induced tissue toxicity, organ damage (mainly in the liver, endocrine organs, and heart), and early death [7].

The introduction of chelating agents capable of removing excessive iron from the body has dramatically increased life expectancy in patients with thalassemia major [8, 9]. Prior to the discovery of DFP, the only option for treatment of iron overload was deferoxamine (DFO), a complex hydroxylamine with high affinity for iron. Its route of administration is critical in achieving the goal of therapy. In fact, due to its high molecular weight and its short half-life (approximately 30 min), it must be administered parenterally (mostly subcutaneously) by prolonged infusion (over 8–12 h) 5–7 nights a week (Thalassemia International Federation Guidelines 2007). The beneficial effects of DFO in preventing early death are well documented [8]. Nevertheless, some patients are unable or unwilling to receive deferoxamine treatment. In countries where it is needed the most, the high costs of the drug and the supplies needed for its administration make it unavailable for most patients. On the other hand, in the Western world, despite the wide accessibility to DFO, some patients do not comply with DFO therapy because of the unpleasant and cumbersome nature of the regime, limiting the usefulness of this chelator [10]. In a

proportion of patients, the low compliance is due to the occurrence of unpleasant local or general side effects, including local reactions at the site of injection, high-frequency hearing loss, visual toxicity, and bone lesions. Consequently, the search for more practical chelators has continued to be a major challenge during the last few decades. Thus the introduction of DFP was accompanied by much hope among hematologists and thalassemia patients alike.

The regulatory approval of Ferriprox in India (1995) and Europe (1999) was a huge step forward in iron overload treatment. Recently, another oral iron chelator, deferasirox (ICL670, Exjade), has been approved for clinical use [11, 12].

Chemistry, Pharmacokinetics, and Pharmacodynamics

DFP is a synthetic analogue of mimosine, an iron chelator isolated from *Mimosa paduca* [13]. DFP has strong iron-binding properties, with a pFe^{3+} of 19.6 and a pFe^{2+} of 5.6, indicating a high degree of relative specificity for the trivalent form of iron. As it is a bidentate iron chelator, three DFP molecules are required to form a complex that occupies the six coordination sites of an iron (Fe^{3+}) atom. Key pharmacologic properties of the compound are shown in figure 1 [13, 14]. As a water-soluble compound having a partition coefficient of 0.11 and with a molecular weight of only 139 Da, it would be expected to move freely through cell membranes throughout the body.

DFP is rapidly and completely absorbed after oral administration, with plasma levels peaking about 1 h after administration and a half-life of 160 min [15]. Foods slow the rate of absorption reducing the peak concentration, with a C_{max} of ~100 μmol/l in the fasting state and ~85 μmol/l when fed [15, 16], but do not significantly reduce the total amount absorbed.

The drug, its compound with iron or its metabolites are excreted in the urine within 3–4 h. A minimal amount of these compounds is excreted in the feces. As DFP is rapidly metabolized by glucuronidation within the liver to its inactive metabolite, it requires thrice-daily administration (overall dose: 75–100 mg/kg) [16].

DFP is available as film-coated, immediate-release tablets containing 500 mg of the active agent and as a palatable liquid formulation containing 100 mg/ml.

DFP Efficacy

Monotherapy

Successful iron chelation therapy depends on the achievement of neutral or negative iron balance, in which the iron excretion equals or exceeds the rate of iron accumulation, which in regularly transfused patients is 0.3–0.5 mg/kg/day. Therefore, the purpose of an effective iron chelation is to prevent or reduce iron accumulation, thus minimizing the risk of iron-induced toxicity. Ideally, this is accomplished by the combined mechanism of excreting excess iron from organs and tissues through the urine and/or feces and inactivating the labile iron. Chelation of labile iron is extremely important since it is highly toxic and, if iron overload is elevated, it is produced 24 h a day. Therefore, for the effective control of labile iron, constant presence of an iron chelator in the body is necessary. By reducing tissue iron stores to levels that can be tolerated by the respective organs, the benefits of a regular transfusion program can be achieved without the deleterious consequences of iron overload.

In transfusion-dependent thalassemia, the greatest source of increased body iron is from the transfused red blood cells (RBC). Transfusion requirements are quite variable depending on the established transfusion regime and blood availability. With the most widely accepted transfusion regime aimed at maintaining the hemoglobin level before transfusion >9–10 g/dl, splenectomized patients usually receive ~120 ml RBC/kg each year, and non-splenectomized patients ~160 ml RBC/kg each year, because of enhanced RBC degradation by an overactive spleen (Thalassemia International Federation Guidelines, 2007). Overall, with this transfusion regime, the total amount of iron received from transfusions would be about 0.3–0.4 mg iron/kg body weight per day.

Measurement of the amount of iron eliminated in urine and feces provides an unequivocal determination of the effectiveness of an iron chelator in removing iron from the body, because normally urine and feces contain negligible amounts of iron (~1 mg/day), except for desquamation of cells (GI and menses) [4]. DFP eliminates iron mainly via urine (about 80%) [16]. Several studies found DFP to have comparable efficacy to subcutaneous DFO in promoting urinary iron excretion [1]. It was found that urinary iron excretion increased with the dose, frequency of administration, and with the degree of iron loading in the patients [16–20]. However, the most comprehensive approach to iron excretion analysis has been carried out by Grady et al. [21], who used full iron balance studies in a metabolic unit to measure total iron output (into feces and urine) compared to the total iron intake (with food and transfusions). These studies demonstrate that 75 mg of DFP/kg/day was comparable to 40 mg of DFO/kg/day and 100 mg of DFP/kg/day was comparable to 60 mg of DFO/kg/day.

Several studies conducted during the 1990s showed that DFP was able to decrease or stabilize body iron, as expressed by sequential serum ferritin or liver iron assessment, despite continual iron treatment with RBC transfusions [22]. Results of randomized clinical trials comparing DFO with DFP demonstrated no difference after 12 months of treatment in serum ferritin levels or liver iron concentration [23, 24]. Similar results have been obtained in other studies [25–27].

Cardiac Profile of DFP

Iron-induced heart failure and arrhythmias are the most common causes of death in patients with thalassemia major, accounting for about 70% of deaths [28]. For this reason, the main role of iron-chelating therapy is to prevent premature death from myocardial iron overload.

Magnetic resonance imaging (MRI), employing the T2* MRI methodology, is the most recent and valuable diagnostic tool to be used in the assessment of cardiac iron load for predicting the risk of iron-induced cardiac damage [29]. T2* MRI is considered the new standard for measuring cardiac iron levels and it has been validated against physical measurements of iron in liver biopsy samples (calibration for heart iron is in progress [Pennell D., pers. commun.; Carpenter and Pennell, pp 146–154, this issue]), and showed high reproducibility with a coefficient of variation of ~5% in multiple sites with different scanners [29, 30]. Anderson et al. [29] found that below a myocardial T2* of 20 ms there was a progressive and significant decline in left ventricular ejection fraction (LVEF). In general, the lower the T2* the higher the risk of cardiac dysfunction, with T2* <8 ms being suggestive of severe iron overload. The effect of different iron chelation therapies on myocardial T2* has been evaluated in a number of studies. Several independent studies have shown that DFP is more effective than DFO in removing cardiac iron. Based on MR T2* and cardiac function, Anderson et al. [31] retrospectively compared myocardial iron content in 15 patients on long-term DFP with 30 matched patients with thalassemia major on long-term DFO. Patients on DFP had significantly higher myocardial T2* (median 34 vs. 11.4 ms; p = 0.02) and higher LVEF than the DFO group (mean 70 ± 6.5 vs. 63 ± 6.9%; p = 0.004). In another retrospective study with more than 4 years of observation, cardiac dysfunction expressed as worsening of preexisting cardiac abnormality or development of new cardiac disease was diagnosed in 4% of the 54 DFP-treated patients and 20% of the 75 DFO-treated patients (p = 0.007) [26]. Several prospective trials have compared the effects of DFP and DFO on myocardial iron. In two studies, DFP at 75 mg/kg/day was as effective as DFO at 50 mg/kg/day for 5–6 days per week at reducing cardiac iron by MR signal intensity ratio [24, 32]. Peng et al. [27] compared cardiac iron, estimated by MR signal intensity and LVEF over 3 years in 13 patients taking DFO (50 mg/kg/day at least 5 days per week) with 11 patients taking DFP (75 mg/kg/day). Cardiac iron was markedly improved in 5 patients on DFP but only in 2 patients on DFO treatment. Patients taking DFP improved their LVEF (from 58.6 ± 6.8 to 65.2 ± 7.1%), whereas there was no significant change in the DFO group (from 63.3 ± 6.3 to 64.6 ± 7.0%). Recently, the most comprehensive results have been obtained in a large, prospective controlled trial, where 61 patients with moderate cardiac iron load (T2* between 10 and 20 ms) previously treated with DFO were randomized to be maintained on DFO (43 mg/kg for 5–7 days per week) or switched to DFP (92 mg/kg/day) [33]. After 6 and 12 months of treatment, they observed a significant improvement in myocardial T2* with both treatments, although the improvement was greater with DFP than DFO [+18 vs. +9% (p = 0.04) at 6 months, and +27 vs. +13% (p = 0.023) at 12 months (p = 0.023)]. LVEF also increased significantly more in the DFP group (3.1 vs. 0.3%; at 12 months, p = 0.003).

A significantly greater cardiac protection with DFP treatment has been reported in a large natural history study performed in Italy, collecting data on survival and causes of death from seven thalassemia centers [34]. The analysis included cardiac events and survival for 359 patients on DFO during the observation period (from

1995 to 2003) and for 157 patients shifted from DFO to DFP at some point during the study period. At baseline, the two groups were comparable regarding age and sex, while serum ferritin was significantly higher in patients switched to DFP (mean serum ferritin 1,860 vs. 1,461 μg/l, p < 0.001). Fifty-two cardiac events, including 10 cardiac deaths, occurred in patients on DFO, whereas DFP-switched patients did not experience any cardiac events.

Overall, the available data show that patients on DFP may have a greater cardiac benefit than DFO-treated patients. The apparently greater efficacy of DFP in removing excess cardiac iron may be related to some physicochemical characteristics of DFP, which facilitate membrane permeation and chelation of intracellular iron: low molecular weight (139 Da compared with 657 Da for DFO), neutral charge, and lipophilicity [35].

Association between DFP and DFO

Looking at the many papers published on the concomitant use of DFP and DFO, a problem of terminology is evident and the term 'combination' has been associated with very different regimes of chelation. However, combination therapy should indicate the assumption of both DFO and DFP treatment on the same day either simultaneously (i.e. DFP taken before breakfast, lunch, and dinner with subcutaneous DFO infusion during the day) or sequentially (i.e. DFP as above with DFO infused during the night). The intensity of this regime can vary according to the severity of iron overload: usually DFP is taken 7 days/week, while subcutaneous DFO infusion varies from 2 to 7 days/week. In patients with heart failure, DFO can be given intravenously to reinforce iron chelation.

Alternate chelation regimes should indicate the days of the week when one or the other chelator is administered.

Combined Chelation

Combination therapy with DFP and DFO was first introduced in 1998 by Wonke et al. [36]. Over the past years, numerous studies have provided data on the efficacy and safety of chelation regimes combining the use of DFP and DFO. The potential advantages of combined chelation are reported in table 1.

Many clinical studies with combination therapy suggest a good control of body iron burden reflected by decreased serum ferritin and, when measured, liver iron concentration [37–40]. However, in these studies very

Table 1. Potential advantages of combination therapy

Different iron pools of chelation
Higher efficacy
Dose decrease → toxicity decrease
Prevention of non-transferrin-bound iron accumulation
Better tolerability
Better compliance
Improvement in quality of life

different combination treatments (i.e. regarding the dose of the two chelators, days of DFO administration, and duration of the study) have been used. A significant improvement in LVEF in comparison with the baseline value has been reported in three papers [38–40]. A randomized, placebo-controlled, double-blind trial suggested that in comparison to the standard chelation monotherapy with DFO, combination therapy with additional DFP reduced myocardial iron (ratio of change in cardiac T2* geometric means 1.50 in combination treatment vs. 1.24 in DFO monotherapy, p = 0.02) and improved absolute LVEF (2.6 vs. 0.6%, p = 0.05) [41].

Several single case reports and a prospective study including 15 patients have demonstrated the efficacy of combined treatment in thalassemia major patients with severe myocardial siderosis and left ventricular dysfunction or heart failure [42–46]. Reversal of heart failure was also observed in a patient with a severe type of juvenile hemochromatosis [47].

Combined DFO and DFP treatment improved several endocrinological complications including glucose metabolism, hypothyroidism, and hypogonadism [48, 49; Farmaki, pers. commun.]. Telfer et al. [50] analyzed survival trends in Cypriot thalassemia major patients before and after 1999, when combination therapy became widespread in Cyprus. They observed that all-cause mortality had increased among the thalassemia population between 1985 and 1999, with a trend toward an increasing proportion of deaths from cardiac-related causes, despite the use of intensive intravenous DFO in individuals at increased risk. With the introduction of combined therapy in 1999, a significant reversal of this trend in mortality for cardiac disease was observed.

Alternate Chelation
The efficacy of an alternating chelation regime has been examined in a prospective, controlled trial where 60 transfusion-dependent thalassemia patients regularly treated with DFO where randomized to continue DFO alone or to receive 5 days/week DFP and 2 days/week DFO for 1 year [51]. In both treatment groups, chelation therapy had similar effects on serum ferritin and liver iron concentration.

More recently, Maggio et al. [52] published the results of a large long-term (5 years of follow-up) multicenter trial, including 213 patients randomized to receive DFO for 4 days/week and DFP for the remaining 3 days/week, or DFP monotherapy for 7 days/week. The trial results showed that there was a significant reduction in serum ferritin levels in the alternating treatment group (p = 0.005). No patients with agranulocytosis were reported in the alternating therapy group compared with 3 patients with agranulocytosis in the DFP-alone group (p = 0.085). Although not statistically significant, these findings suggest that during alternate treatment the risk of agranulocytosis may be lower than with DFP monotherapy.

In another multicenter, long-term, randomized, controlled trial, Maggio et al. [53] compared DFO versus DFP alone, alternate or combined DFO-DFP iron chelation treatments in 265 patients with thalassemia major. No deaths occurred with DFP alone, or combined treatment; 1 death occurred with alternate DFO-DFP treatment, whereas 10 deaths occurred with the DFO treatment.

Clinical Safety Profile

Long-term studies in a large number of patients who participated in a DFP clinical development program and the extensive postmarketing use provided well-documented data on the DFP safety profile [52–55] (ApoPharma postmarketing surveillance program). These data have demonstrated that long-term therapy is not associated with an increase in frequency or severity of adverse drug reactions (ADR) compared with those reported in the short-term clinical studies. The safety data have also shown that ADR with DFP are well characterized, predictable, and usually reversible, provided that the patients are closely monitored.

GI symptoms, such as nausea, vomiting, and abdominal pain, are the most frequently reported DFP-related ADR. In a long-term prospective study which monitored 187 patients with thalassemia major, GI symptoms occurred overall in 33% of patients in the 1st year, decreasing to 3% in subsequent years [54]. In general, these events were mild/moderate in intensity and resolved within 1 week of onset without discontinuation of therapy in most patients. Despite the high frequency, only a restricted number of patients discontinued therapy because of GI complaints. Similar results have been reported in other studies [24, 55, 56]. About 5% of patients report increased appetite considered related to DFP, but its significance is unknown. The new liquid DFP formulation showed a lower incidence of GI adverse reactions (vomiting 6% of the patients, abdominal pain 6%, and nausea 1%) than with the tablet formulation [57].

Joint symptoms (pain and/or swelling) were associated with the use of DFP in 3.9–20% [54–56, 58]. The frequency of arthropathy seems to increase with the severity of iron overload. In a clinical study, joint problems have been reported in 9% of patients with baseline serum ferritin <2,500 μg/l and in 26% of the patients with baseline ferritin >5,000 μg/l during the 1st year of treatment [59]. However, the association between high serum ferritin and joint symptoms was not sustained in the extension up to 4 years of this study [54]. A particularly high incidence of arthropathy has been reported in Indian patients treated with DFP (up to 41%), which has been attributed to the severe iron overload or undefined ethnic genetic background [60]. Joint symptoms, sometimes associated with myalgia, are mild/moderate in most patients and generally resolved without discontinuation of therapy. However, in some patients, joint symptoms may be severe enough to warrant temporary or permanent interruption of the drug or reduction of the dose. Overall, about 2% of the patients discontinued DFP because of joint symptoms. Unlike GI problems, which usually manifest in the first weeks of treatment, joint problems may occur even after years of treatment. Antinuclear antibody titers, rheumatoid factor, anti-double-stranded DNA, and anti-histone antibodies were assessed at baseline and then sequentially at 3-month intervals for 1 year in a large clinical study; the levels indicate that the episodes of arthropathy were not associated with an autoimmune disease [59]. Increase in serum alanine aminotransferase (ALT) activity was reported in about 7% of the patients particularly in the first months of treatment. The transient, asymptomatic, and usually mild changes in ALT levels and the absence of a progressive increase over time have been reported in several studies [24, 54, 56, 58]. However, it is recommend that serum ALT levels be monitored at regular intervals and DFP interruption or dose reduction should be considered if a persistent increase in serum ALT occurs. Overall, 1% of patients discontinued DFP for severe ALT increase in clinical trials.

In 1998, DFP use was associated with an increase in liver fibrosis in 5 of 14 patients [61]. However, an editorial accompanying the report outlined that the design of the study, the small liver biopsy samples, and the lack of an appropriate control group precluded any definitive conclusion [62]. A separate blind review of the same 14 biopsies did not confirm the original results [63]. Since then, several studies conducted to evaluate liver histology changes during therapy with DFP did not show any evidence of DFP-induced liver fibrosis [64–66]. Three independent pathologists analyzed the largest collection of liver biopsies (116 samples) from 56 patients treated with DFP for a mean of 3.1 years and demonstrated no evidence of progression of liver fibrosis that may be attributed to DFP toxicity [67].

Low plasma zinc levels have been reported in patients treated with DFP, particularly in those with diabetes mellitus. In long-term controlled studies, a slight decrease in plasma zinc has been observed over time, but the mean value remained within the normal reference range [54]. Overall, low plasma zinc levels are not a common problem in patients treated with DFP, but periodic monitoring can be suggested especially in patients with diabetes.

Reddish discoloration of urine due to excretion of the chromophore iron-DFP complex has been reported in some patients treated with DFP [59].

Embryotoxicity and teratogenicity have been reported in non-iron-loaded animals after DFP administration [68]. Therefore, women of child-bearing age should be counseled to avoid pregnancy and use proper contraception methods while on DFP therapy. In case of pregnancy, DFP should be immediately discontinued. However, few uneventful pregnancies with healthy newborns have been reported [69–71]. DFP should also be avoided in breast-feeding mothers. No significant abnormalities have been found in newborns from those pregnancies carried to term in partners of patients taking DFP [72].

The most serious ADR associated with DFP use is agranulocytosis, defined as a confirmed (i.e. in two consecutive counts) absolute neutrophil count (ANC) <0.5 × 10^9/l. It occurred in about 1% of the patients (0.2–0.3 episodes per 100 patient-years) in controlled studies [54, 55, 59]. Agranulocytosis has been reported most commonly within the 1st year of treatment (median 159 days). One episode which occurred after 9 years of treatment could be attributed to the concomitant medications received by the patient for the treatment of chronic hepatitis C. Agranulocytosis usually resolves with interruption of DFP, but sometimes treatment with G-CSF may be needed for faster recovery. The median duration reported is 9 days (range 3–85). Fatal outcome due to severe infections associated with DFP-related agranulocytosis has

Table 2. Recommendations for monitoring DFP-treated patients for the most common ADR

ADR	Assessment	Frequency
Neutropenia/agranulocytosis	white blood cell count (ANC)	5–10 days
Increased liver enzymes	ALT	at least quarterly
GI and joint problems	report to physician	at symptom onset

been reported in some patients [73, 74]. To detect early signs of agranulocytosis, weekly (5–10 days) ANC monitoring is recommended for all patients treated with DFP. Patients should be advised to immediately interrupt DFP at the first sign of neutropenia/agranulocytosis and to report to their physician any symptom indicative of infection.

Episodes of milder neutropenia (defined as a confirmed ANC between 0.5 and 1.5 $\times$ 10^9/l) have been reported in 3.6–8.5% of the patients [54–56, 59]. This condition is usually reversible on discontinuation of the drug. The mechanism of DFP-related agranulocytosis is unknown and studies are in progress to identify potential genetic risk factors. It appears that the mechanism for agranulocytosis and milder neutropenia may be different. Neutropenia occurs significantly more often in non-splenectomized patients and in association with viral infections [59]. Because of the risk of recurrence, reintroduction of DFP after an initial episode of agranulocytosis is not recommended.

Table 2 offers recommendations for monitoring the most relevant ADR during DFP therapy.

New Potential Indications for DFP

A growing body of evidence suggests that local iron misdistribution in subcellular organelles without body iron overload may play some role in neurodegenerative diseases such as Friedreich ataxia, pantothenate kinase neurodegeneration, Huntington's disease, Parkinson's disease, and Alzheimer's disease [75, 76]. Therefore, iron chelators may have a valuable potential therapeutic approach in these conditions.

Boddaert et al. [77] assessed the possibility of reducing brain iron accumulation in patients with Friedreich ataxia, using regimes of DFP suitable for patients with no systemic iron overload. The rationale was to use a membrane-permeant chelator for removing labile iron from brain cell organelles, hence reducing iron-dependent free-radical formation and tissue damage. A 6-month DFP treatment with 20–30 mg/kg/day of 9 adolescent patients reduced neuropathy and ataxic gait in the youngest patients. Brain MRI showed a reduction in R2*, specifically dentate nuclei, indicating a reduction in regional iron accumulation. A phase II, randomized, placebo-controlled trial in Europe, Australia, and Canada investigating the safety, tolerability, and efficacy of DFP in patients with Friedreich ataxia is in progress. Regression of symptoms after selective iron chelation with DFP has also been reported in a case of neurodegeneration with brain iron accumulation [78].

Conclusion

DFP seems to be an effective oral iron chelator which is able to reduce iron overload and maintain safe levels of body iron assessed by serum ferritin and liver concentrations. Moreover, DFP monotherapy or DFP-DFO combination therapy have greater efficacy than DFO alone in reducing excess cardiac iron levels, improving cardiac function assessed by MRI, reducing iron-induced cardiac morbidity, and consequently in improving survival.

DFP has a well-known long-term safety profile. Adverse reactions to DFP are usually controllable and reversible following appropriate monitoring.

References

1 Kontoghiorghes GJ, Aldouri MA, Sheppard L, Hoffbrand AV: 1,2-Dimethyl-3-hydroxy-pyrid-4-one, an orally active chelator for treatment of iron overload. Lancet 1987;i: 1294–1295.
2 Kontoghiorghes GJ: New orally active iron chelators. Lancet 1985;i:817.
3 Hoffbrand AV: Deferiprone therapy for transfusional iron overload. Best Pract Res Clin Haematol 2005;18:299–317.
4 Andrews NC: Disorders of iron metabolism. N Engl J Med 1999;341:1986–1995.

5 Hershko C, Graham G, Bates GW, Rachmilewitz EA: Non-specific serum iron in thalassaemia: an abnormal serum iron fraction of potential toxicity. Br J Haematol 1978; 40:255–263.

6 Cabantchik ZI, Breuer W, Zanninelli G, Cianciulli P: LPI-labile plasma iron in iron overload. Best Pract Res Clin Haematol 2005; 18:277–287.

7 Rund D, Rachmilewitz E: Beta-thalassemia. N Engl J Med 2005;353:1135–1146.

8 Olivieri NF, Nathan DG, MacMillan JH, Wayne AS, Liu PP, McGee A, Martin M, Koren G, Cohen AR: Survival in medically treated patients with homozygous β-thalassemia. N Engl J Med 1994;331:574–578.

9 Borgna-Pignatti C, Rugolotto S, De Stefano P, Zhao H, Cappellini MD, Del Vecchio GC, Romeo MA, Forni GL, Gamberini MR, Ghilardi R, Piga A, Cnaan A: Survival and complications in patients with thalassemia major treated with transfusion and deferoxamine. Haematologica 2004;89:1187–1193.

10 Cunningham MJ, Macklin EA, Neufeld EJ, Cohen AR: Complications of beta-thalassemia major in North America. Blood 2004; 104:34–39.

11 Cappellini MD, Cohen A, Piga A, Bejaoui M, Perrotta S, Agaoglu L, Aydinok Y, Kattamis A, Kilinc Y, Porter J, Capra M, Galanello R, Fattoum S, Drelichman G, Magnano C, Verissimo M, Athanassiou-Metaxa M, Giardina P, Kourakli-Symeonidis A, Janka-Schaub G, Coates T, Vermylen C, Olivieri N, Thuret I, Opitz H, Ressayre-Djaffer C, Marks P, Alberti D: A phase 3 study of deferasirox (ICL670), a once-daily oral iron chelator, in patients with beta-thalassemia. Blood 2006; 107:3455–3462.

12 Galanello R, Piga A, Forni GL, Bertrand Y, Foschini ML, Bordone E, Leoni G, Lavagetto A, Zappu A, Longo F, Maseruka H, Hewson N, Sechaud R, Belleli R, Alberti D: Phase II clinical evaluation of deferasirox, a once-daily oral chelating agent, in pediatric patients with beta-thalassemia major. Haematologica 2006;91:1343–1351.

13 Clarke ET, Martell AE: Stabilities of 1,2-dimethyl-3-hydroxy-4-pyridinone chelates of divalent and trivalent metal ions. Inorg Chim Acta 1992;191:57–63.

14 Tam TF, Leung-Toung R, Li W, Wang Y, Karimian K, Spino M: Iron chelator research: past, present, and future. Curr Med Chem 2003;10:983–995.

15 Matsui D, Klein J, Hermann C, Grunau V, McClelland R, Chung D, St-Louis P, Olivieri N, Koren G: Relationship between the pharmacokinetics and iron excretion pharmacodynamics of the new oral iron chelator 1,2-dimethyl-3-hydroxypyrid-4-one in patients with thalassemia. Clin Pharmacol Ther 1991; 50:294–298.

16 Al-Refaie FN, Sheppard LN, Nortey P, Wonke B, Hoffbrand AV: Pharmacokinetics of the oral iron chelator deferiprone (L1) in patients with iron overload. Br J Haematol 1995;89:403–408.

17 Kontoghiorghes GJ, Aldouri MA, Hoffbrand AV, Barr J, Wonke B, Kourouclaris T, Sheppard L: Effective chelation of iron in beta thalassaemia with the oral chelator 1,2-dimethyl-3-hydroxypyrid-4-one. Br Med J (Clin Res Ed) 1987;295:1509–1512.

18 Kontoghiorghes GJ, Bartlett AN, Hoffbrand AV, Goddard JG, Sheppard L, Barr J, Nortey P: Long-term trial with the oral iron chelator 1,2-dimethyl-3-hydroxypyrid-4-one (L1). I. Iron chelation and metabolic studies. Br J Haematol 1990;76:295–300.

19 Agarwal MB, Gupte SS, Viswanathan C, Vasandani D, Ramanathan J, Desai N, Puniyani RR, Chhablani AT: Long-term assessment of efficacy and safety of L1, an oral iron chelator, in transfusion dependent thalassaemia: Indian trial. Br J Haematol 1992; 82:460–466.

20 Collins AF, Fassos FF, Stobie S, Lewis N, Shaw D, Fry M, Templeton DM, McClelland RA, Koren G, Olivieri NF: Iron-balance and dose-response studies of the oral iron chelator 1,2-dimethyl-3-hydroxypyrid-4-one (L1) in iron-loaded patients with sickle cell disease. Blood 1994;83:2329–2333.

21 Grady RW, Berdoukas VA, Rachhmilewitz EA, Galanello R, Borgna-Pignatti C, Ladis V, Sitarou M, Hadjigavriel M, Giardina PJ: Exploring the shuttle effect: implications for combined chelator treatment (abstract). Santorini, Proc 12th Int Conf Oral Chelation in the Treatment of Thalassemia and Other Diseases, 2002, pp 62–63.

22 Hoffbrand AV, Cohen A, Hershko C: Role of deferiprone in chelation therapy for transfusional iron overload. Blood 2003;102:17–24.

23 Olivieri NF, Koren G, Hermann C, Bentur Y, Chung D, Klein J, St Louis P, Freedman MH, McClelland RA, Templeton DM: Comparison of oral iron chelator L1 and desferrioxamine in iron-loaded patients. Lancet 1990; 336:1275–1279.

24 Maggio A, D'Amico G, Morabito A, Capra M, Ciaccio C, Cianciulli P, Di Gregorio F, Garozzo G, Malizia R, Magnano C, Mangiagli A, Quarta G, Rizzo M, D'Ascola DG, Rizzo A, Midiri M: Deferiprone versus deferoxamine in patients with thalassemia major: a randomized clinical trial. Blood Cells Mol Dis 2002;28:196–208.

25 Taher A, Sheikh-Taha M, Koussa S, Inati A, Neeman R, Mourad F: Comparison between deferoxamine and deferiprone (L1) in iron-loaded thalassemia patients. Eur J Haematol 2001;67:30–34.

26 Piga A, Gaglioti C, Fogliacco E, Tricta F: Comparative effects of deferiprone and deferoxamine on survival and cardiac disease in patients with thalassemia major: a retrospective analysis. Haematologica 2003;88:489–496.

27 Peng CT, Chow KC, Chen JH, Chiang YP, Lin TY, Tsai CH: Safety monitoring of cardiac and hepatic systems in beta-thalassemia patients with chelating treatment in Taiwan. Eur J Haematol 2003;70:392–397.

28 Borgna-Pignatti C, Rugolotto S, De Stefano P, Zhao H, Cappellini MD, Del Vecchio GC, Romeo MA, Forni GL, Gamberini MR, Ghilardi R, Piga A, Cnaan A: Survival and complications in patients with thalassemia major treated with transfusion and deferoxamine. Haematologica 2004;89:1187–1193.

29 Anderson LJ, Holden S, Davis B, Prescott E, Charrier CC, Bunce NH, Firmin DN, Wonke B, Porter J, Walker JM, Pennell DJ: Cardiovascular T2-star (T2*) magnetic resonance for the early diagnosis of myocardial iron overload. Eur Heart J 2001;22:2171–2179.

30 Westwood MA, Anderson LJ, Firmin DN, Gatehouse PD, Lorenz CH, Wonke B, Pennell DJ: Interscanner reproducibility of cardiovascular magnetic resonance T2* measurements of tissue iron in thalassemia. J Magn Reson Imaging 2003;18:616–620.

31 Anderson LJ, Wonke B, Prescott E, Holden S, Walker JM, Pennell DJ: Comparison of effects of oral deferiprone and subcutaneous desferrioxamine on myocardial iron concentrations and ventricular function in beta-thalassaemia. Lancet 2002;360:516–520.

32 Galia M, Midiri M, Bartolotta V, Morabito A, Rizzo M, Mangiagli A, Malizia R, Borsellino Z, Capra M, D'Ascola DG, Magnano C, Gerardi C, Rigano P, Maggio A: Potential myocardial iron content evaluation by magnetic resonance imaging in thalassemia major patients treated with deferoxamine or deferiprone during a randomized multicenter prospective clinical study. Hemoglobin 2003;27:63–76.

33 Pennell DJ, Berdoukas V, Karagiorga M, Ladis V, Piga A, Aessopos A, Gotsis ED, Tanner MA, Smith GC, Westwood MA, Wonke B, Galanello R: Randomized controlled trial of deferiprone or deferoxamine in beta-thalassemia major patients with asymptomatic myocardial siderosis. Blood 2006;107:3738–3744.

34 Borgna-Pignatti C, Cappellini MD, De Stefano P, Del Vecchio GC, Forni GL, Gamberini MR, Ghilardi R, Piga A, Romeo MA, Zhao H, Cnaan A: Cardiac morbidity and mortality in deferoxamine- or deferiprone-treated patients with thalassemia major. Blood 2006; 107:3733–3737.

35 Hider RC, Liu ZD: Emerging understanding of the advantage of small molecules such as hydroxypyridinones in the treatment of iron overload. Curr Med Chem 2003;10:1051–1064.

36 Wonke B, Wright C, Hoffbrand AV: Combined therapy with deferiprone and desferrioxamine. Br J Haematol 1998;103:361–364.

37 Mourad FH, Hoffbrand AV, Sheikh-Taha M, Koussa S, Khoriaty AI, Taher A: Comparison between desferrioxamine and combined therapy with desferrioxamine and deferiprone in iron overloaded thalassaemia patients. Br J Haematol 2003;121:187–189.

38 Origa R, Bina P, Agus A, Crobu G, Defraia E, Dessì C, Leoni G, Muroni PP, Galanello R: Combined therapy with deferiprone and desferrioxamine in thalassemia major. Haematologica 2005;90:1309–1314.

39 Kattamis A, Kassou C, Berdousi H, Ladis V, Papassotiriou I, Kattamis C: Combined therapy with desferrioxamine and deferiprone in thalassemic patients: effect on urinary iron excretion. Haematologica 2003;88:1423–1425.

40 Daar S, Pathare AV: Combined therapy with desferrioxamine and deferiprone in beta thalassemia major patients with transfusional iron overload. Ann Hematol 2006;85:315–319.

41 Tanner MA, Galanello R, Dessi C, Smith GC, Westwood MA, Agus A, Roughton M, Assomull R, Nair SV, Walker JM, Pennell DJ: A randomized, placebo-controlled, double-blind trial of the effect of combined therapy with deferoxamine and deferiprone on myocardial iron in thalassemia major using cardiovascular magnetic resonance. Circulation 2007;115:1876–1884.

42 Wu KH, Chang JS, Tsai CH, Peng CT: Combined therapy with deferiprone and desferrioxamine successfully regresses severe heart failure in patients with beta-thalassemia major. Ann Hematol 2004;83:471–473.

43 Tsironi M, Deftereos S, Andriopoulos P, Farmakis D, Meletis J, Aessopos A: Reversal of heart failure in thalassemia major by combined chelation therapy: a case report. Eur J Haematol 2005;74:84–85.

44 Porcu M, Landis N, Salis S, Corda M, Orrù P, Serra E, Usai B, Matta G, Galanello R: Effects of combined deferiprone and desferrioxamine iron chelating therapy in beta-thalassemia major end-stage heart failure: a case report. Eur J Heart Fail 2007;9:320–322.

45 Tavecchia L, Masera N, Russo P, Cirò A, Vincenzi A, Vimercati C, Masera G: Successful recovery of acute hemosiderotic heart failure in beta-thalassemia major treated with a combined regimen of desferrioxamine and deferiprone. Haematologica 2006;91(6 suppl):ECR19.

46 Tanner MA, Galanello R, Dessi C, Smith GC, Westwood MA, Agus A, Pibiri M, Nair SV, Walker JM, Pennell DJ: Combined chelation therapy in thalassemia major for the treatment of severe myocardial siderosis with left ventricular dysfunction. J Cardiovasc Magn Reson 2008;10:12.

47 Fabio G, Minonzio F, Delbini P, Bianchi A, Cappellini MD: Reversal of cardiac complications by deferiprone and deferoxamine combination therapy in a patient affected by a severe type of juvenile hemochromatosis (JH). Blood 2007;109:362–364.

48 Farmaki K, Angelopoulos N, Anagnostopoulos G, Gotsis E, Rombopoulos G, Tolis G: Effect of enhanced iron chelation therapy on glucose metabolism in patients with beta-thalassaemia major. Br J Haematol 2006;134:438–444.

49 Christoforidis A, Perifanis V, Athanassiou-Metaxa M: Combined chelation therapy improves glucose metabolism in patients with beta-thalassaemia major. Br J Haematol 2006;135:271–272.

50 Telfer P, Coen PG, Christou S, Hadjigavriel M, Kolnakou A, Pangalou E, Pavlides N, Psiloines M, Simamonian K, Skordos G, Sitarou M, Angastiniotis M: Survival of medically treated thalassemia patients in Cyprus. Trends and risk factors over the period 1980–2004. Haematologica 2006;91:1187–1192.

51 Galanello R, Kattamis A, Piga A, Fischer R, Leoni G, Ladis V, Voi V, Lund U, Tricta F: A prospective randomized controlled trial on the safety and efficacy of alternating deferoxamine and deferiprone in the treatment of iron overload in patients with thalassemia. Haematologica 2006;91:1241–1243.

52 Maggio A, Vitrano A, Capra M, Cuccia L, Gagliardotto F, Filosa A, Romeo MA, Magnano C, Caruso V, Argento C, Gerardi C, Campisi S, Violi P, Malizia R, Cianciulli P, Rizzo M, D'Ascola DG, Quota A, Prossomariti L, Fidone C, Rigano P, Pepe A, D'Amico G, Morabito A, Gluud C: Long-term sequential deferiprone-deferoxamine versus deferiprone alone for thalassaemia major patients: a randomized clinical trial. Br J Haematol 2009;145:245–254.

53 Maggio A, Vitrano A, Capra M, Cuccia L, Gagliardotto F, Filosa A, Magnano C, Rizzo M, Caruso V, Gerardi C, Argento C, Campisi S, Cantella F, Commendatore F, D'Ascola DG, Fidone C, Ciancio A, Galati MC, Giuffrida G, Cingari R, Giugno G, Lombardo T, Prossomariti L, Malizia R, Meo A, Roccamo G, Romeo MA, Violi P, Cianciulli P, Rigano P: Improving survival with deferiprone treatment in patients with thalassemia major: a prospective multicenter randomised clinical trial under the auspices of the Italian Society for Thalassemia and Hemoglobinopathies. Blood Cells Mol Dis 2009;42:247–251.

54 Cohen AR, Galanello R, Piga A, De Sanctis V, Tricta F: Safety and effectiveness of long-term therapy with the oral iron chelator deferiprone. Blood 2003;102:1583–1587.

55 Ceci A, Baiardi P, Felisi M, Cappellini MD, Carnelli V, De Sanctis V, Galanello R, Maggio A, Masera G, Piga A, Schettini F, Stefàno I, Tricta F: The safety and effectiveness of deferiprone in a large-scale, 3-year study in Italian patients. Br J Haematol 2002;118:330–336.

56 Al-Refaie FN, Hershko C, Hoffbrand AV, Kosaryan M, Olivieri NF, Tondury P, Wonke B: Results of long-term deferiprone (L1) therapy: a report by the International Study Group on Oral Iron Chelators. Br J Haematol 1995;91:224–229.

57 El-Beshlawi A, Sari TT, Chan LL, Tricta F, El-Alfy M: The safety and efficacy of an oral solution formulation of deferiprone in children with transfusional iron overload (abstract). Singapore, 11th International Conference on Thalassaemia and hemoglobinopathies and 13th International TIF Conference for Thalassaemia Patients and Parents, October 8–11, 2008.

58 Olivieri NF, Brittenham GM, Matsui D, Berkovitch M, Blendis LM, Cameron RG, McClelland RA, Liu PP, Templeton DM, Koren G: Iron-chelation therapy with oral deferiprone in patients with thalassemia major. N Engl J Med 1995;332:918–922.

59 Cohen AR, Galanello R, Piga A, Dipalma A, Vullo C, Tricta F: Safety profile of the oral iron chelator deferiprone: a multicentre study. Br J Haematol 2000;108:305–312.

60 Choudhry VP, Pati HP, Saxena A, Malaviya AN: Deferiprone, efficacy and safety. Indian J Pediatr 2004;71:213–216.

61 Olivieri NF, Brittenham GM: Long-term trials of deferiprone in Cooley's anemia. Ann NY Acad Sci 1998;850:217–222.

62 Kowdley KV, Kaplan MM: Iron-chelation therapy with oral deferiprone – toxicity or lack of efficacy? N Engl J Med 1998;339:468–469.

63 Callea F: Iron chelation with oral deferiprone in patients with thalassemia. N Engl J Med 1998;339:1710–1711.

64 Hoffbrand AV, AL-Refaie F, Davis B, Siritanakatkul N, Jackson BF, Cochrane J, Prescott E, Wonke B: Long-term trial of deferiprone in 51 transfusion-dependent iron overloaded patients. Blood 1998;91:295–300.

65 Piga A, Longo F, Voi V, Facello S, Miniero R, Dresow B: Late effects of bone marrow transplantation for thalassemia. Ann NY Acad Sci 1998;850:294–299.

66 Galanello R, De Virgiliis S, Agus A: Sequential liver fibrosis grading during deferiprone treatment in patients with thalassemia major (abstract). Hamburg, 9th International Conference on Oral Chelation in the Treatment of Thalassaemia and Other Diseases, March 25–28, 1999, p 50.

67 Wanless IR, Sweeney G, Dhillon AP, Guido M, Piga A, Galanello R, Gamberini MR, Schwartz E, Cohen AR: Lack of progressive hepatic fibrosis during long-term therapy with deferiprone in subjects with transfusion-dependent beta-thalassemia. Blood 2002;100:1566–1569.

68 Berdoukas V, Bentley P, Frost H, Schnebli HP: Toxicity of oral iron chelator L1. Lancet 1993;341:1088.

69 Goudsmit R, Kersten MJ: Long-term treatment of transfusion hemosiderosis with the oral iron chelator L1. Drugs Today 1992;28:133–135.

70 Kersten MJ, Lange R, Smeets ME, Vreugdenhil G, Roozendaal KJ, Lameijer W, Goudsmit R: Long-term treatment of transfusional iron overload with the oral iron chelator deferiprone (L1): a Dutch multicenter trial. Ann Hematol 1996;73:247–252.

71 Gogtay JA, Agarwal MB: Clinical experience with Kelfer (deferiprone) in India over the last 12 years (abstract). Santorini, 12th International Conference on Oral Chelation in the Treatment of Thalassemia and Other Diseases, 2002, p 89.

72 Magnano C, Caruso V, Caruso M, Anastasi S: Two cases of healthy children born thalassemic patients treated with L1. Bangkok, 7th International Conference on Thalassemia and the Haemoglobinopathies, 1999.

73 Müller A, Soyano A, Soyano-Müller A: Irreversible aplastic anemia after treatment with deferiprone in a patient with blackfan diamond anemia and hemochromatosis (abstract). Blood 2000;96:13b.

74 Apotex Research: Ferriprox: Periodic Safety Update Report, PSUR. Toronto, Apotex, 2003.

75 Whitnall M, Richardson DR: Iron: a new target for pharmacological intervention in neurodegenerative diseases. Semin Pediatr Neurol 2006;13:186–197.

76 Molina-Holgado F, Hider RC, Gaeta A, Williams R, Francis P: Metals ions and neurodegeneration. Biometals 2007;20:639–654.

77 Boddaert N, Le Quan Sang KH, Rötig A, Leroy-Willig A, Gallet S, Brunelle F, Sidi D, Thalabard JC, Munnich A, Cabantchik ZI: Selective iron chelation in Friedreich ataxia: biologic and clinical implications. Blood 2007;110:401–408.

78 Forni GL, Balocco M, Cremonesi L, Abbruzzese G, Parodi RC, Marchese R: Regression of symptoms after selective iron chelation therapy in a case of neurodegeneration with brain iron accumulation. Mov Disord 2008;23:904–907.

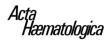

Acta Haematol 2009;122:165–173
DOI: 10.1159/000243801

Published online: November 10, 2009

Deferasirox (Exjade®) for the Treatment of Iron Overload

M.D. Cappellini[a]   A. Taher[b]

[a]Fondazione Ospedale Maggiore Policlinico, Istituto di Ricovero e Cura a Carattere Scientifico, Università di Milano, Milano, Italia; [b]American University Beirut, Beirut, Lebanon

Key Words

Chelation · Deferasirox · Myelodysplastic syndromes · Pediatric anemia · Sickle cell disease · Thalassemia

Abstract

Deferasirox is a once-daily oral iron chelator with established dose-dependent efficacy in both adult and pediatric patients with transfusional iron overload. The clinical development program has demonstrated the efficacy of deferasirox for up to 4.5 years of treatment in patients with various underlying anemias, including β-thalassemia, myelodysplastic syndromes, sickle cell disease, aplastic anemia, and other rare anemias. In addition to reducing key indicators of total body iron levels (serum ferritin, liver iron concentration, and toxic labile plasma iron), deferasirox has also demonstrated the ability to remove cardiac iron and prevent future cardiac iron accumulation. Emerging long-term data confirm the tolerability profile of deferasirox, and data on patient compliance render deferasirox a suitable therapeutic option for patients with chronic conditions requiring ongoing iron chelation therapy. Data continue to accumulate in a wide range of patient groups, including those with non-transfusion-dependent anemias such as hereditary hemochromatosis.

Copyright © 2009 S. Karger AG, Basel

Introduction

Long-term red blood cell transfusion for the treatment of various chronic anemias inevitably leads to the accumulation of iron in the body. Several iron chelators have been developed, designed to mobilize tissue iron by forming complexes that are excreted in the feces and/or urine. Deferoxamine (Desferal®; DFO; Novartis Pharma, Basel, Switzerland) was developed more than 40 years ago and the wealth of clinical experience in iron-overloaded patients has established a role for iron chelators in the improvement of patient quality of life and overall survival [1, 2]. However, due to its poor oral bioavailability and short plasma half-life, subcutaneous administration is required 5–7 days/week, often resulting in poor compliance [3]. Deferiprone (Ferriprox®; Apotex, Toronto, Ont., Canada) was the first oral iron chelator available in the European Union and a number of countries outside the USA and Canada for the second-line treatment of iron overload in adult patients with β-thalassemia in whom DFO therapy is contraindicated or inadequate (European Medicines Agency). Deferiprone has a short half-life (3–4 h) and therefore requires three-times daily dosing. Deferasirox (Exjade®; Novartis Pharma) was developed as a once-daily oral iron chelator through a rational drug development program and represents a new class of tridentate iron chelators. Deferasirox is currently approved in

Prof. Maria Domenica Cappellini
Fondazione Policlinico, IRCCS, Università di Milano
Via F. Sforza 35
IT–20122 Milano (Italy)
Tel. +39 02 5503 3358, Fax +39 347 788 5455, E-Mail maria.cappellini@unimi.it

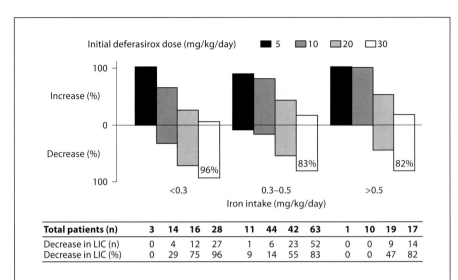

Total patients (n)	3	14	16	28	11	44	42	63	1	10	19	17
Decrease in LIC (n)	0	4	12	27	1	6	23	52	0	0	9	14
Decrease in LIC (%)	0	29	75	96	9	14	55	83	0	0	47	82

Fig. 1. Impact of transfusional iron intake and deferasirox dose on LIC. (This research was originally published by Cohen et al. [12] in *Blood.*)

many countries worldwide for the treatment of chronic iron overload due to blood transfusions in patients aged ≥2 years. The efficacy and safety of deferasirox has been evaluated in patients with β-thalassemia and also in a wide range of patients with other underlying anemias, including myelodysplastic syndromes (MDS), sickle cell disease (SCD), aplastic anemia (AA), Diamond-Blackfan anemia (DBA), and various other rare anemias [3–11].

Thalassemia

The symptoms of β-thalassemia major occur as a result of complete or partial reduction in the production of the β-globin protein (due to mutations in the β-globin gene) that constitutes part of functional hemoglobin. This results in ineffective erythropoiesis and hemolysis causing severe life-threatening anemia, which normally presents in the 1st year of life and can be fatal during infancy or childhood if untreated. Red blood cell transfusions are the primary treatment approach and are often required from early childhood.

Deferasirox Therapy in Patients with β-Thalassemia Major

The pharmacokinetic profile of oral deferasirox was established in patients with β-thalassemia in two small, randomized, double-blind, placebo-controlled, dose-finding studies [3, 4]. The pharmacokinetic profile, in particular the observed half-life for deferasirox (11–19 h), was sup-

portive of a once-daily dosing regimen as deferasirox plasma levels were maintained within the therapeutic range over a 24-hour period providing continuous chelation coverage [4]. Deferasirox 20 mg/kg/day was also identified as an effective oral dose and shown to be generally well tolerated [3]. Furthermore, deferasirox 20–30 mg/kg/day was shown to be as effective in reducing liver iron concentration (LIC) as DFO at a dose of 40 mg/kg/day [10]. Additional analyses of these data demonstrated that ongoing transfusional iron loading affects the response to deferasirox and, together with serum ferritin trends, needs to be monitored on an ongoing basis and used to guide deferasirox dosing in order to achieve individual patient therapeutic goals of either maintenance or reduction in iron load (fig. 1) [8, 12]. This approach was evaluated in the EPIC (Evaluation of Patients' Iron Chelation) trial where the deferasirox dose was titrated every 3 months according to serum ferritin trends and safety markers [7]. Data from a large group (n = 937) of regularly transfused patients with β-thalassemia major showed that changes in serum ferritin were reflective of dose adjustments and mean iron intake during treatment. Patients who received an average actual dose ≥30 mg/kg/day had the greatest reduction in serum ferritin (–962 ng/ml; p < 0.0001 vs. baseline) and patients receiving <20 or ≥20–<30 mg/kg/day maintained their iron balance [13]. In a retrospective analysis including a large number of patients with β-thalassemia, doses >30 mg/kg/day were shown to safely reduce serum ferritin, which is important for heavily transfused patients who may require higher deferasirox doses to reduce body iron burden [14]. As well as affecting serum ferritin levels and LIC, deferasirox can also reduce levels of labile plasma iron (LPI) in patients with β-thalassemia major. LPI is a directly chelatable form of non-transferrin-bound iron readily taken up by cells and is able to participate in redox cycling reactions resulting in the formation of harmful reactive oxygen species [15, 16]. Deferasirox doses ≥20 mg/kg/day provided sustained reduction in LPI levels and may therefore contribute to a reduction in unregulated tissue iron loading [17, 18].

Long-term data are critical for the evaluation of iron chelation therapy in patients with β-thalassemia due to the chronic nature of the disease. Median follow-up of patients treated with deferasirox has now been reported in extended phase trials for up to 4.5 years. Results have confirmed that the efficacy of deferasirox depends on both dose and transfusion [19, 20] even in patients unsuccessfully chelated with DFO and/or deferiprone due to unacceptable toxicity, poor response to therapy or non-compliance with treatment regimens [21].

Tolerability and Management of Adverse Events in Patients with β-Thalassemia

The most common drug-related (investigator-assessed) adverse events (AEs) identified in β-thalassemia patients are abdominal pain, nausea, diarrhea, vomiting, and rash; however, the annual frequency of these AEs has generally been shown to decrease from year to year [20]. Such AEs are clinically manageable with regular patient monitoring as the many deferasirox clinical studies have provided information on their onset, severity, duration, and frequency. For diarrhea, patients should be advised to stay hydrated and take an anti-diarrheal for up to 2 days if required. Patients may also benefit from taking deferasirox in the evening rather than the morning or adding products such as Lactaid to their diet [22]. Mild-to-moderate skin rashes are likely to resolve spontaneously; however, severe cases may require dose interruptions and/or adjustments [22]. Non-progressive increases in serum creatinine (rising above the mean of measurements before treatment by >33% on two consecutive occasions) have been observed in approximately one third of patients treated with deferasirox [8]. However, these increases were dose dependent and often resolved spontaneously. It is recommended that serum creatinine levels are assessed in duplicate before therapy begins and monthly thereafter with any significant increases managed by dose reductions and/or interruptions [22, 23].

Patient Preferences

Compliance with iron chelation therapy is an important issue for patients, as with many chronic conditions. Patients need to be educated about the risks of iron overload and the benefits of remaining compliant with therapy. As deferasirox is an oral therapy, it may be expected that patient compliance would be superior to that seen with DFO infusions [6]. Assessment of patient preferences demonstrated satisfaction and convenience with deferasirox therapy as compared with DFO, with 97% of patients with β-thalassemia who switched to deferasirox from DFO preferring deferasirox. Patients preferred deferasirox due to convenience (37%), absence of injection site soreness (25%) and less disruption to their day (23%) [24]. Greater satisfaction and convenience with deferasirox may translate into improvements in patient compliance and increased effectiveness of chelation therapy.

Deferasirox Therapy in Pediatric Patients with β-Thalassemia

The efficacy and safety of deferasirox have been evaluated in pediatric β-thalassemia patients as young as 2 years of age. The pharmacokinetic profile of deferasirox in pediatric patients (aged 2–7 years) also supports a once-daily dosing regimen; however, the steady-state exposure to deferasirox in children and adolescents is ~20–30% lower than in adults [4, 9]. A conservative dosing strategy was used in preliminary trials in children resulting in an overall gradual increase in LIC [9]; 10 mg/kg/day was used irrespective of the degree of iron overload at baseline with dose adjustments allowed only after 12 weeks of treatment. Longer-term follow-up data in pediatric patients treated with deferasirox for up to 5 years have now demonstrated a dose-dependent reduction in iron burden [25, 26].

The safety profile of deferasirox in pediatric patients is similar to that of adult patients during the 5-year follow-up at doses of up to 30 mg/kg/day [25, 26]. The recommended starting dose and dosing modifications are the same for pediatric and adult patients [23]. To date, neither progressive renal, hepatic, or bone marrow dysfunctions nor deferasirox-induced negative impacts on growth and sexual development have been reported [26].

Deferasirox Therapy in β-Thalassemia Patients with Cardiac Siderosis

Iron-induced cardiac failure and arrhythmia are responsible for as many as 71% of deaths in patients with

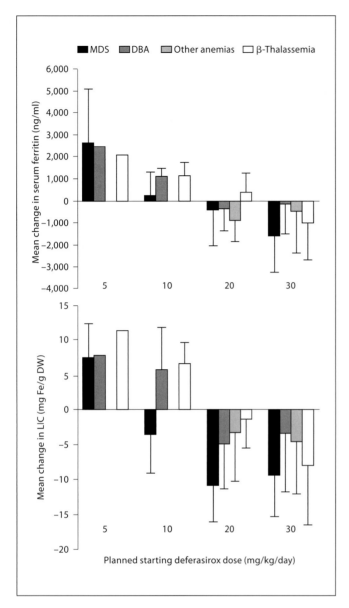

Fig. 2. Deferasirox is effective in reducing serum ferritin and LIC across a range of transfusion-dependent anemias. Other anemias include AA (n = 5), α-thalassemia (n = 3), sideroblastic anemia (n = 3), myelofibrosis (n = 2), pure red cell aplasia (n = 2), pyruvate kinase deficiency (n = 2), autoimmune hemolytic anemia (n = 1), Fanconi's anemia (n = 1), hereditary sideroblastic anemia (n = 1), erythropenia (n = 1), and unspecified anemia (n = 1). DW = Dry weight.

β-thalassemia major [1, 27]. The ability of deferasirox to remove iron from the heart is therefore of particular interest. Initial studies in animal models demonstrating the efficacy of deferasirox to reduce cardiac iron content [28] were followed by clinical data to support the effi-

cacy of deferasirox in the removal of cardiac iron and prevention of myocardial siderosis in patients with β-thalassemia major [29–32]. After 1 year of deferasirox treatment (mean dose: 32.6 mg/kg/day) in 114 patients with baseline myocardial T2* of 20 ms (indicative of cardiac iron accumulation), myocardial T2* was shown to improve significantly from a geometric mean baseline of 11.2 to 12.9 ms while left ventricular ejection fraction was maintained at ~67% [30]. In a cohort of 78 patients with normal myocardial iron levels (T2* >20 ms), myocardial T2* was maintained after treatment with deferasirox for 1 year (32.0 ms at baseline and 32.5 ms after 12 months of therapy at a mean dose of 27.6 mg/kg/day), left ventricular ejection fraction significantly increased from 67.7 to 69.6% (p < 0.0001) and body iron burden as assessed by serum ferritin and LIC were significantly reduced [32].

Iron Chelation Therapy in Patients with Thalassemia Intermedia

Defects in the β-globin gene may also result in a diagnosis of β-thalassemia intermedia, which has a wide clinical spectrum with patients often remaining asymptomatic until adult life [33]. In contrast to patients with β-thalassemia major, thalassemia intermedia patients are rarely transfusion dependent; however, they are susceptible to gradual iron overload through increased intestinal absorption of iron secondarily due to chronic anemia and decreased serum hepcidin caused by GDF15 overexpression, which may be exacerbated by occasional blood transfusions. Therefore patients need to be assessed for iron overload. Cardiac iron loading appears to be less of an issue in patients with thalassemia intermedia [34]; however, iron overload should still be monitored in both the liver and the heart. As the clinical consequences of iron overload in thalassemia intermedia are the same as in transfused patients with β-thalassemia major, patients may benefit from iron chelation therapy. Few studies have assessed chelation therapy in thalassemia intermedia [35, 36]; however, there is an ongoing 1-year trial of deferasirox in >150 patients with thalassemia intermedia, representing the first large-scale study of an iron-chelating agent in this patient population.

Myelodysplastic Syndromes

MDS is a group of heterogeneous disorders characterized by impaired blood cell production by the bone marrow. Managing MDS is often complicated by the gener-

Table 1. Efficacy of deferasirox across a variety of transfusion-dependent anemias included in the EPIC trial

	All patients (n = 1,744) [7]	β-Thalassemia major (n = 937) [13]	MDS (n = 341) [43]	AA (n = 116) [45]	Rare anemias (n = 43) [46]	DBA (n = 14) [47]
Baseline serum ferritin, ng/ml	3,135	3,157	2,730	3,254	3,161	2,289
Median change in serum ferritin, ng/ml	–264	–129	–253	–964	–832	–790
p value	<0.0001	0.0007	0.0019	0.0003	0.0275	0.0121
Average deferasirox dose during study, mg/kg/day	22.2	24.2	19.2	17.6	18.6	21.0

ally advanced age of patients (median age 65–70 years) [37]. Red blood cell transfusions are the mainstay of supportive care for MDS [38] and up to 90% of MDS patients with chronic anemia become dependent on transfusions to manage the symptoms of anemia [38]; however, blood transfusion therapy is associated with increased risk of iron toxicity. Chelation therapy is recommended by several treatment guidelines in patients who have an International prognostic Scoring System risk of low or intermediate-1 and serum ferritin levels of >1,000–2,000 ng/ml, depending on transfusion requirements [37, 39, 40]. Response to chelation therapy may not be the same as in β-thalassemia patients due to differences in the magnitude of directly chelatable iron pools, and thus specific data are required to evaluate efficacy and safety [5]. There are a limited number of small-scale studies on the use of DFO and deferiprone in this patient population; however, several larger clinical trials with deferasirox have provided more robust data [5, 41–43].

Deferasirox Therapy in Patients with MDS
Deferasirox has been shown to maintain or reduce body iron in patients with MDS in several clinical trials [5, 42–44]. In one study of 176 patients, deferasirox decreased mean serum ferritin over 1 year and normalized LPI levels [42]. In another study comparing responses to iron chelation among various disease groups, a similar pattern of dose-dependent iron excretion was observed in patients with MDS compared with β-thalassemia (fig. 2) [5]. More recently, the EPIC trial enrolled the largest cohort of MDS patients to date (n = 341). Despite a high transfusion requirement and iron burden in this cohort, almost 50% had received no prior chelation therapy. Deferasirox provided significant reduction in serum ferritin over the 1-year treatment period with appropriate dose adjustments every 3 months as required (table 1) [7, 13, 43, 45–47]. The most common AEs con-

sidered related to treatment included mild-to-moderate gastrointestinal symptoms consistent with those identified in patients with β-thalassemia. However, the discontinuation rate was higher and investigations are ongoing to determine possible contributing factors such as existing co-morbidities and the advanced age of this patient subgroup [43].

Sickle Cell Disease

SCD is a group of inherited disorders caused by the sickle mutation affecting the β-globin chain of hemoglobin. Erythrocytes containing hemoglobin S have irregular morphology and under low oxygen conditions, hemoglobin S polymerizes leading to 'sickled' cells [48]. The pathogenesis of SCD relates to the shortened lifespan of the sickled erythrocytes (16–20 days in contrast to a lifespan of 120 days for normal erythrocytes) and adhesion of the sickled erythrocytes to the microvascular endothelium. Transfusion of red blood cells on a chronic or intermittent basis is therefore important in the management of SCD. There is increasing evidence of the value of transfusions particularly in reducing the risk of stroke in pediatric patients with SCD [49, 50]. However, progressive iron loading and tissue injury as a result of frequent blood transfusions appear to be similar to those in other transfusion populations [51].

Deferasirox Therapy in Patients with SCD
In comparison with DFO, deferasirox has been shown to have similar efficacy and a well-defined, manageable safety profile in both adult and pediatric patients (aged 3–54 years) with SCD [6]. After 1 year of treatment with deferasirox (10–30 mg/kg/day), LIC was significantly reduced compared with baseline (p < 0.05) and serum ferritin was also decreased, although with intrapatient vari-

ability. The incidence of AEs including sickle cell crisis was also similar in both groups (46.2% with deferasirox and 42.9% with DFO) [6]. As part of this phase II study, patient-reported outcomes were also evaluated. Throughout the study, significantly more patients receiving deferasirox reported being 'satisfied' or 'very satisfied' with treatment compared with those on DFO (p < 0.001) [52]. Similar outcomes were also reported regarding convenience of deferasirox therapy. Cumulative 3.5-year data of deferasirox in SCD patients have now demonstrated continued reduction in body iron (based on serum ferritin levels) without any exposure-associated increased risk of AEs, renal dysfunction, or progressive increases in serum creatinine [53].

Other Rare Anemias

Deferasirox Therapy in Patients with DBA

DBA is a rare type of congenital erythroid aplasia that occurs in 5–10 of every 1 million births, where anemia occurs due to the failure of erythropoiesis [54]. In a 1-year study of deferasirox in patients with DBA, doses of 20 and 30 mg/kg/day induced a negative iron balance in a similar pattern to patients with other underlying anemias such as β-thalassemia and MDS (fig. 1; n = 30) [5]. These data were supported by results from the prospective EPIC trial, where a significant reduction in serum ferritin from baseline was observed in patients with DBA receiving an average daily dose of ≥20–<30 mg/kg/day (–1,095.0 ng/ml; p = 0.0015; table 1) [47]. The majority of DBA patients (86%) in the EPIC trial had received prior chelation therapy with DFO and/or deferiprone; however, median baseline serum ferritin was still elevated. The AE profile was similar to that observed in other patient groups [5, 47].

Deferasirox Therapy in Patients with AA

AA often results from other bone marrow disorders (such as MDS) as a result of complete bone marrow failure. The worldwide annual incidence is estimated at 2 of every 1,000,000 births [55]. AA can be treated with bone marrow transplantation or immunosuppressive therapy; however, the main supportive therapy involves regular blood transfusions [56]. Over a 1-year treatment period, deferasirox significantly reduced iron burden in patients with AA at an average actual dose of 17.6 ± 4.8 mg/kg/day (table 1) [45]. Interestingly, 68% of AA patients enrolled in this trial had received no prior treatment with chelation therapy even though they had an elevated median serum ferritin at baseline (3,254 ng/ml) associated with significant negative outcomes [1], thereby indicating a need for iron chelation therapy in this patient population [45]. Deferasirox was generally well tolerated, with the most common (>10%) drug-related AEs including nausea, diarrhea, and rash; most AEs (>95%) were of mild-to-moderate severity.

Future Developments

To date, the deferasirox clinical development program has focused on the treatment of patients with transfusional iron overload; however, a wider perspective is now being taken with the investigation of deferasirox in a number of other conditions including hereditary hemochromatosis (HH; characterized by progressive iron overloading through increased intestinal absorption [57]), chronic hepatitis C [58], porphyria cutanea tarda (a common type of porphyria which can be associated with hemochromatosis [59]), and mucormycosis.

Phlebotomy is the standard of care in HH patients to reduce serum ferritin levels and prevent clinical complications of iron overload. However, compliance with phlebotomy tends to decrease with time due to the inconvenience of frequent clinic visits and discomfort of the procedure; some patients may also be poor candidates due to underlying medical disorders and/or poor venous access. A study is ongoing to evaluate the safety and efficacy of deferasirox as a further treatment option in patients with HH (adult patients homozygous for the C282Y mutation) [60] and preliminary results suggest that deferasirox doses of 5, 10 and 15 mg/kg/day are effective at reducing iron burden with an acceptable safety profile [61]. Preliminary studies in the treatment of chronic hepatitis C infection with interferon/ribavirin have suggested that previous treatment with deferasirox may improve early viral response rates [58]. A pilot trial to investigate the efficacy and tolerability of deferasirox in the treatment of porphyria cutanea tarda is currently recruiting patients (ClinicalTrials.gov identifier: NCT00599326). Deferasirox has also been shown to significantly improve survival and decrease tissue fungal burden in mice infected with mucormycosis [62]. A clinical study to determine whether the addition of deferasirox to standard antifungal therapy, liposomal amphotericin B (LAmB; AmBisome), is safe and effective for the treatment of mucormycosis is also currently recruiting patients (DEFEAT Mucor study; ClinicalTrials.gov identifier: NCT00419770).

Additionally, the benefits of reduced iron levels in bone marrow transplant patients before and after transplantation have been recognized [63] and, therefore, deferasirox also has a potential application in this patient population.

Conclusions

Long-term red blood cell transfusions are required for the treatment of many anemias including β-thalassemia, MDS, SCD, DBA, and AA. Frequent transfusions inevitably lead to iron overload, which has serious clinical sequelae. The oral iron chelator deferasirox has been evaluated in heterogeneous populations of patients with a variety of underlying anemias demonstrating consistent efficacy and safety profiles. The results from the large-scale EPIC trial and data from long-term studies further support these observations as well as the importance of timely dose adjustments based on serum ferritin trends to adapt therapy for individual patients. Emerging data on the cardiac efficacy of deferasirox are also encouraging in both the prevention and treatment of cardiac iron accumulation. Deferasirox therefore represents a significant advance in the treatment of a wide variety of patients with chronic iron overload, with further potential applications still to be explored.

Acknowledgments

Financial support for medical editorial assistance was provided by Novartis Pharmaceuticals. We thank Dr. Rebecca Helson for medical editorial assistance.

References

1 Olivieri NF, Nathan DG, MacMillan JH, Wayne AS, Liu PP, McGee A, Martin M, Koren G, Cohen AR: Survival in medically treated patients with homozygous β-thalassemia. N Engl J Med 1994;331:574–578.

2 Olivieri NF, Brittenham GM: Iron-chelating therapy and the treatment of thalassemia. Blood 1997;89:739–761.

3 Nisbet-Brown E, Olivieri NF, Giardina PJ, Grady RW, Neufeld EJ, Séchaud R, Krebs-Brown AJ, Anderson JR, Alberti D, Sizer KC, Nathan DG: Effectiveness and safety of ICL670 in iron-loaded patients with thalassaemia: a randomised, double-blind, placebo-controlled, dose-escalation trial. Lancet 2003;361:1597–1602.

4 Galanello R, Piga A, Alberti D, Rouan MC, Bigler H, Sechaud R: Safety, tolerability, and pharmacokinetics of ICL670, a new orally active iron-chelating agent in patients with transfusion-dependent iron overload due to beta-thalassemia. J Clin Pharmacol 2003;43:565–572.

5 Porter J, Galanello R, Saglio G, Neufeld EJ, Vichinsky E, Cappellini MD, Olivieri N, Piga A, Cunningham MJ, Soulières D, Gattermann N, Tchernia G, Maertens J, Giardina P, Kwiatkowski J, Quarta G, Jeng M, Forni GL, Stadler M, Cario H, Debusscher L, Della Porta M, Cazzola M, Greenberg P, Alimena G, Rabault B, Gathmann I, Ford JM, Alberti D, Rose C: Relative response of patients with myelodysplastic syndromes and other transfusion-dependent anaemias to deferasirox (ICL670): a 1-year prospective study. Eur J Haematol 2008;80:168–176.

6 Vichinsky E, Onyekwere O, Porter J, Swerdlow P, Eckman J, Lane P, Files B, Hassell K, Kelly P, Wilson F, Bernaudin F, Forni GL, Okpala I, Ressayre-Djaffer C, Alberti D, Holland J, Marks P, Fung E, Fischer R, Mueller BU, Coates T: A randomized comparison of deferasirox versus deferoxamine for the treatment of transfusional iron overload in sickle cell disease. Br J Haematol 2007;136:501–508.

7 Cappellini MD, El-Beshlawy A, Kattamis A, Lee JW, Seymour JF, Li CK, Habr D, Domokos G, Hmissi A, Elalfy MS: Efficacy and safety of deferasirox (Exjade®) in patients with transfusion-dependent anemias: 1-year results from the large, prospective, multicenter EPIC study (abstract). Blood 2008;112:3875.

8 Cappellini MD, Cohen A, Piga A, Bejaoui M, Perrotta S, Agaoglu L, Aydinok Y, Kattamis A, Kilinc Y, Porter J, Capra M, Galanello R, Fattoum S, Drelichman G, Magnano C, Verissimo M, Athanassiou-Metaxa M, Giardina B, Kourakli-Symeonidis A, Janka-Schaub G, Coates T, Vermylen C, Olivieri N, Thuret I, Opitz H, Ressayre-Djaffer C, Marks P, Alberti D: A phase 3 study of deferasirox (ICL670), a once-daily oral iron chelator, in patients with β-thalassemia. Blood 2006;107:3455–3462.

9 Galanello R, Piga A, Forni GL, Bertrand Y, Foschini ML, Bordone E, Leoni G, Lavagetto A, Zappu A, Longo F, Maseruka H, Hewson N, Sechaud R, Belleli R, Alberti D: Phase II clinical evaluation of deferasirox, a once-daily oral chelating agent, in pediatric patients with β-thalassemia major. Haematologica 2006;91:1343–1351.

10 Piga A, Galanello R, Forni GL, Cappellini MD, Origa R, Zappu A, Donato G, Bordone E, Lavagetto A, Zanaboni L, Sechaud R, Hewson N, Ford JM, Opitz H, Alberti D: Randomized phase II trial of deferasirox (Exjade®, ICL670), a once-daily, orally-administered iron chelator, in comparison to deferoxamine in thalassemia patients with transfusional iron overload. Haematologica 2006;91:873–880.

11 Taher A, El-Beshlawy A, Elalfy MS, Al Zir K, Daar S, Damanhouri G, Habr D, Kriemler-Krahn U, Hmissi A, Al Jefri A: Efficacy and safety of deferasirox, an oral iron chelator, in heavily iron-overloaded patients with β-thalassaemia: the ESCALATOR study. Eur J Haematol 2009;82:458–465.

12 Cohen AR, Glimm E, Porter JB: Effect of transfusional iron intake on response to chelation therapy in β-thalassemia major. Blood 2008;111:583–587.

13 Cappellini MD, Elalfy MS, Kattamis A, Seymour JF, Lee Lee C, Porter JB, El-Beshlawy A, Habr D, Domokos G, Hmissi A, Taher A: Efficacy and safety of once-daily, oral iron chelator deferasirox (Exjade®) in a large group of regularly transfused patients with β-thalassemia major (abstract). Blood 2008;112:3878.

14 Cappellini MD, Taher A, Vichinsky E, Galanello R, Piga A, Lawniczek T, Jehl V, Rojkjaer L, Porter JB: Efficacy and tolerability of deferasirox doses >30 mg/kg/day in patients with transfusion-dependent anaemia and iron overload (abstract). Haematologica 2008;93(suppl 1):845.

15 Porter J: Pathophysiology of iron overload. Hematol Oncol Clin North Am 2005;19 (suppl 1):7–12.

16 Esposito BP, Breuer W, Sirankapracha P, Pootrakul P, Hershko C, Cabantchik ZI: Labile plasma iron in iron overload: redox activity and susceptibility to chelation. Blood 2003;102:2670–2677.

17 Daar S, Pathare A, Nick H, Kriemler-Krahn U, Hmissi A, Habr D, Taher A: Reduction in labile plasma iron during treatment with deferasirox, a once-daily oral iron chelator, in heavily iron-overloaded patients with β-thalassaemia. Eur J Haematol 2009;82:454–457.

18 Porter JB, Cappellini MD, El-Beshlawy A, Kattamis A, Seymour JF, Lee JW, Nick H, Habr D, Domokos G, Hmissi A, Taher A: Effect of deferasirox (Exjade®) on labile plasma iron levels in heavily iron-overloaded patients with transfusion-dependent anemias enrolled in the large-scale, prospective 1-year EPIC trial (abstract). Blood 2008;112:3881.

19 Cappellini MD, Vichinsky E, Galanello R, Piga A, Williamson P, Porter JB: Long-term treatment with deferasirox (Exjade®, ICL670), a once-daily oral iron chelator, is effective in patients with transfusion-dependent anemias (abstract). Blood 2007;110:2777.

20 Cappellini MD, Galanello R, Piga A, Cohen A, Kattamis A, Aydinok Y, Williamson P, Rojkjaer L, Porter JB: Efficacy and safety of deferasirox (Exjade®) with up to 4.5 years of treatment in patients with thalassemia major: a pooled analysis (abstract). Blood 2008; 112:5411.

21 Taher A, El-Beshlawy A, Elalfy MS, Al Zir K, Daar S, Damanhouri G, Habr D, Kriemler-Krahn U, Hmissi A, Al Jefri A: Efficacy and safety of once-daily oral deferasirox (Exjade®) during a median of 2.7 years of treatment in heavily iron-overloaded patients with β-thalassemia (abstract). Blood 2008; 112:5409.

22 Vichinsky E: Clinical application of deferasirox: Practical patient management. Am J Hematol 2008;83:398–402.

23 Exjade (deferasirox) Prescribing Information. Novartis Pharmaceuticals Corporation. http://www.pharma.us.novartis.com/product/pi/exjade.pdf.

24 Cappellini MD, Bejaoui M, Agaoglu L, Porter J, Coates T, Jeng M, Lai ME, Mangiagli A, Strauss G, Girot R, Watman N, Ferster A, Loggetto S, Abish S, Cario H, Zoumbos N, Vichinsky E, Opitz H, Ressayre-Djaffer C, Abetz L, Rofail D, Baladi JF: Prospective evaluation of patient-reported outcomes during treatment with deferasirox or deferoxamine for iron overload in patients with β-thalassemia. Clin Ther 2007;29:909–917.

25 Piga A, Forni GL, Kattamis A, Kattamis C, Aydinok Y, Rodriguez M, Rojkjaer L, Galanello R: Deferasirox (Exjade®) in pediatric patients with β-thalassemia: update of 4.7-year efficacy and safety from extension studies (abstract). Blood 2008;112:3883.

26 Piga A, Kebaili K, Galanello R, Jehl V, Rebischung C, Maseruka H, Rojkjaer L, Forni GL: Cumulative efficacy and safety of 5-year deferasirox (Exjade®) treatment in pediatric patients with thalassemia major: a phase II multicenter prospective trial (abstract). Blood 2008;112:5413.

27 Zurlo MG, De Stefano P, Borgna-Pignatti C, Di Palma A, Piga A, Melevendi C, Di Gregorio F, Burattini MG, Terzoli S: Survival and causes of death in thalassaemia major. Lancet 1989;ii:27–30.

28 Wood JC, Otto-Duessel M, Gonzales I, Aguilar MI, Shimada H, Nick H, Nelson M, Moats R: Deferasirox and deferiprone remove cardiac iron in the iron-overloaded gerbil. Transl Res 2006;148:272–280.

29 Garbowski M, Eleftheriou P, Pennell D, Tanner M, Porter JB: Impact of compliance, ferritin and LIC on long-term trends in myocardial T2* with deferasirox (abstract). Blood 2008;112:116.

30 Pennell D, Porter JB, Cappellini MD, Li CK, Aydinok Y, Lee Lee C, Kattamis A, Smith G, Habr D, Domokos G, Hmissi A, Taher A: Efficacy and safety of deferasirox (Exjade®) in reducing cardiac iron in patients with β-thalassemia major: results from the cardiac substudy of the EPIC trial (abstract). Blood 2008;112:3873.

31 Wood JC, Thompson AA, Paley C, Kang B, Giardina P, Harmatz P, Virkus J, Coates TD: Deferasirox (Exjade®) monotherapy significantly reduces cardiac iron burden in chronically transfused β-thalassemia patients: an MRI T2* study (abstract). Blood 2008;112:3882.

32 Pennell D, Sutcharitchan P, El-Beshlawy A, Aydinok Y, Taher A, Smith G, Habr D, Kriemler-Krahn U, Hmissi A, Porter JB: Efficacy and safety of deferasirox (Exjade®) in preventing cardiac iron overload in β-thalassemia patients with normal baseline cardiac iron: results from the cardiac substudy of the EPIC trial (abstract). Blood 2008;112:3874.

33 Taher A, Isma'eel H, Cappellini MD: Thalassemia intermedia: revisited. Blood Cells Mol Dis 2006;37:12–20.

34 Origa R, Barella S, Argiolas GM, Bina P, Agus A, Galanello R: No evidence of cardiac iron in 20 never or minimally transfused patients with thalassemia intermedia. Haematologica 2008;93:1095–1096.

35 Cossu P, Toccafondi C, Vardeu F, Sanna G, Frau F, Lobrano R, Cornacchia G, Nucaro A, Bertolino F, Loi A, De Virgiliis S, Cao A: Iron overload and desferrioxamine chelation therapy in beta-thalassemia intermedia. Eur J Pediatr 1981;137:267–271.

36 Olivieri NF, Koren G, Matsui D, Liu PP, Blendis L, Cameron R, McClelland RA, Templeton DM: Reduction of tissue iron stores and normalization of serum ferritin during treatment with the oral iron chelator L1 in thalassemia intermedia. Blood 1992;79: 2741–2748.

37 National Comprehensive Cancer Network. NCCN Clinical Practice Guidelines in Oncology v.2: Myelodysplastic Syndromes. http://www.nccn.org/professionals/physician_gls/pdf/mds.pdf.

38 Hellström-Lindberg E: Management of anemia associated with myelodysplastic syndrome. Semin Hematol 2005;42(suppl 1): S10–S13.

39 Bennett JM: Consensus statement on iron overload in myelodysplastic syndromes. Am J Hematol 2008;83:858–861.

40 Gatterman N: Iron overload in myelodysplastic syndromes. Hematol Oncol Clin North Am 2005;19(suppl 1):1–26.

41 Min YH, Kim HJ, Lee KH, Yoon SS, Lee JH, Park HS, Kim JS, Kim HY, Shim H, Seong CM, Kim CS, Chung J, Hyun MS, Jo DY, Jung CW, Sohn SK, Yoon HJ, Kim BS, Joo YD, Park CY, Cheong JW: A multi-center, open label study evaluating the efficacy of iron chelation therapy with deferasirox in transfusional iron overload patients with myelodysplastic syndromes or aplastic anemia using quantitative R₂ MRI (abstract). Blood 2008;112:3649.

42 List AF, Baer MR, Steensma D, Raza A, Esposito J, Virkus J, Paley C, Feigert J, Besa EC: Iron chelation with deferasirox (Exjade®) improves iron burden in patients with myelodysplastic syndromes (MDS) (abstract). Blood 2008;112:634.

43 Gattermann N, Schmid M, Della Porta M, Taylor K, Seymour JF, Habr D, Domokos G, Hmissi A, Guerci-Bresler A, Rose C: Efficacy and safety of deferasirox (Exjade®) during 1 year of treatment in transfusion-dependent patients with myelodysplastic syndromes: results from EPIC trial (abstract). Blood 2008;112:633.

44 Greenberg PL, Schiffer C, Koller CA, Glynos T, Paley C: Change in liver iron concentration (LIC), serum ferritin (SF) and labile plasma iron (LPI) over 1 year of deferasirox (DFX/Exjade®) therapy in a cohort of myelodysplastic patients (abstract). Blood 2008; 112:5083.

45 Lee JW, Yoon SS, Shen ZX, Hsu HC, Ganser A, Habr D, Domokos G, Hmissi A, Porter JB: Iron chelation in regularly transfused patients with aplastic anemia: efficacy and safety results from the large deferasirox EPIC trial (abstract). Blood 2008;112:439.

46 Porter JB, Lin KH, Habr D, Domokos G, Hmissi A, Thein SL: Deferasirox efficacy and safety for the treatment of transfusion-dependent iron overload in patients with a range of rare anemias (abstract). Blood 2008; 112:1419.

47 Porter JB, Forni GL, Beris P, Taher A, Habr D, Domokos G, Hmissi A, Cappellini MD: Efficacy and safety of 1 year's treatment with deferasirox (Exjade®): assessment of regularly transfused patients with Diamond-Blackfan anemia enrolled in the EPIC study (abstract). Blood 2008;112:1048.

48 Claster S, Vichinsky EP: Managing sickle cell disease. Br Med J 2003;327:1151–1155.

49 Adams RJ, McKie VC, Hsu L, Files B, Vichinsky E, Pegelow C, Abboud M, Gallagher D, Kutlar A, Nichols FT, Bonds DR, Brambilla D: Prevention of a first stroke by transfusions in children with sickle cell anemia and abnormal results on transcranial Doppler ultrasonography. N Engl J Med 1998;339:5–11.

50 Adams RJ, Brambilla D: Discontinuing prophylactic transfusions used to prevent stroke in sickle cell disease. N Engl J Med 2005;353:2769–2778.

51 Vichinsky E, Butensky E, Fung E, Hudes M, Theil E, Ferrell L, Williams R, Louie L, Lee PD, Harmatz P: Comparison of organ dysfunction in transfused patients with SCD or β thalassemia. Am J Hematol 2005;80:70–74.

52 Vichinsky E, Pakbaz Z, Onyekwere O, Porter J, Swerdlow P, Coates T, Lane P, Files B, Mueller BU, Coic L, Forni GL, Fischer R, Marks P, Rofail D, Abetz L, Baladi JF: Patient-reported outcomes of deferasirox (Exjade®, ICL670) versus deferoxamine in sickle cell disease patients with transfusional hemosiderosis: substudy of a randomized open-label phase II trial. Acta Haematol 2008;119:133–141.

53 Vichinsky E, Coates T, Thompson AA, Bernaudin F, Rodriguez M, Rojkjaer L, Heeney MM: Deferasirox (Exjade®), the once-daily oral iron chelator, demonstrates safety and efficacy in patients with sickle cell disease (SCD): 3.5-year follow-up (abstract). Blood 2008;112:1420.

54 Diamond Blackfan Anemia Support Group. Diamond Blackfan Anemia Syndrome. http://www.cafamily.org.uk/Direct/d27.html.

55 Risks of agranulocytosis and aplastic anemia. A first report of their relation to drug use with special reference to analgesics. The International Agranulocytosis and Aplastic Anemia Study. JAMA 1986;256:1749–1757.

56 Marsh JC, Ball SE, Darbyshire P, Gordon-Smith EC, Keidan AJ, Martin A, McCann SR, Mercieca J, Oscier D, Roques AW, Yin JAL: Guidelines for the diagnosis and management of acquired aplastic anaemia. Br J Haematol 2003;123:782–801.

57 Beutler E: Iron storage disease: facts, fiction and progress. Blood Cells Mol Dis 2007;39:140–147.

58 Goubran HA, Essmat G, Morcos HH, Amin SN: Pilot results: pre-treatment with deferasirox increases the chances of rapid viral response in patients with chronic hepatitis C infection treated with PEG-interferon/ribavirin (abstract). Blood 2007;110:2281.

59 Kostler E, Wollina U: Therapy of porphyria cutanea tarda. Expert Opin Pharmacother 2005;6:377–383.

60 Pietrangelo A, Brissot P, Bonkovsky H, Niederau C, Rojkjaer L, Weitzman R, Bodner J, Bailey S, Phatak PD: Design of an ongoing phase I/II open-label, dose-escalation trial using the oral chelator deferasirox to treat iron overload in HFE-related hereditary hemochromatosis (HH) (abstract). Blood 2007;110:2680.

61 Pietrangelo A, Brissot P, Bonkovsky H, Niederau C, Rojkjaer L, Weitzman R, Williamson P, Schoenborn-Kellenberger O, Phatak P: A phase I/II, open-label, dose-escalation trial using the once-daily oral chelator deferasirox to treat iron overload in HFE-related hereditary hemochromatosis. J Hepatol 2009, submitted.

62 Ibrahim AS, Gebermariam T, Fu Y, Lin L, Husseiny MI, French SW, Schwartz J, Skory CD, Edwards JE Jr, Spellberg BJ: The iron chelator deferasirox protects mice from mucormycosis through iron starvation. J Clin Invest 2007;117:2649–2657.

63 Jastaniah W, Harmatz P, Pakbaz Z, Fischer R, Vichinsky E, Walters MC: Transfusional iron burden and liver toxicity after bone marrow transplantation for acute myelogenous leukemia and hemoglobinopathies. Pediatr Blood Cancer 2008;50:319–324.

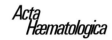

Acta Haematol 2009;122:174–183
DOI: 10.1159/000243802

Published online: November 10, 2009

Iron Metabolism and Iron Chelation in Sickle Cell Disease

Patrick B. Walter   Paul Harmatz   Elliott Vichinsky

Children's Hospital & Research Center Oakland, Oakland, Calif., USA

Key Words

Cytokines · Iron metabolism · Iron trafficking ·
Non-transferrin-bound iron · Pediatric hemoglobinopathy ·
Sickle cell disease · Transfusion

Abstract

This review highlights recent advances in iron metabolism that are relevant to sickle cell disease (SCD). SCD is a common hemoglobinopathy that results in chronic inflammation. Improved understanding of how iron metabolism is controlled by proteins such as hepcidin, ferroportin, hypoxia-inducible factor 1, and growth differentiation factor 15 have revealed how they are involved in the organ toxicity of SCD. SCD patients have lower levels of non-transferrin-bound iron (NTBI) relative to other hemoglobinopathies, such as thalassemia. Care for SCD now commonly uses transfusion that results in iron overload and necessitates the need for chelation. New oral chelation therapy using deferasirox (Exjade/ICL670) appears to be safe and may even lower the amount of toxic free NTBI and enhance patient compliance. Finally, we suggest that iron metabolism and trafficking is different in SCD compared to other hemoglobinopathies. The high levels of inflammatory cytokines in SCD may enhance macrophage/reticuloendothelial cell iron and/or renal cell iron retention. This makes the tissues that retain iron different in SCD, and thus the organs that fail in SCD are different from those of other hemoglobinopathies, such as the cardiomyopathy or endocrinopathies of thalassemia.

Copyright © 2009 S. Karger AG, Basel

Introduction

Historical Perspective of Sickle Cell Disease

Sickle cell disease (SCD) is one of the most common hemoglobinopathies and was first recognized in West Africa possibly in 1670 in a Ghanaian family [1]. However, it was only first reported in the African medical literature in the 1870s likely because the symptoms were similar to other tropical diseases in Africa and not usually examined. Most of the earliest descriptive reports of the disease involved black patients in the US with the first report of SCD in 1910 by James B. Herrick [85].

Pathophysiology of SCD

SCD is a very common world health problem with several thousand affected births each year [2], and it is hematologically characterized by sickle-shaped erythrocytes. The first molecular elucidation of the sickling by Pauling and colleagues revealed that hemoglobin from SCD patients has a different electrophoretic mobility compared to normal hemoglobin [86]. This was later shown to be caused by a point mutation in the second nucleotide of the sixth codon of the β-globin chain, causing a substitution of valine for glutamic acid, resulting in hemoglobin S. Patients with SCD have at least one of the two β-hemoglobin subunits replaced with hemoglobin S. This review will focus on iron metabolism in the homozygous state (Hb SS) of SCD. While historical work showed that sickling only occurs in deoxygenated erythrocytes, more recent molecular studies have shown that

Elliott Vichinsky
Children's Hospital and Research Center Oakland
747 52nd Street
Oakland, CA 94609 (USA)
Tel. +1 510 428 3885, Fax +1 510 450 5813, E-Mail evichinsky@mail.cho.org

sickle hemoglobin interacts between the β6 valine and complementary regions of adjacent hemoglobin molecules. The interaction forms highly ordered polymers that distort the shape of the erythrocytes, making them stiff and poorly deformable, which leads to blockage and microvascular hypoxia-reperfusion cycles. SCD hemoglobin can also bind to the erythrocyte membrane and act as a Fenton reagent, increasing the generation of oxidants such as superoxide and hydroxyl radicals [3]. Other sources of oxidants unique to the SCD vasculature include xanthine oxidase released from the liver, nitric oxide and secondary oxides of nitrogen [4] and endothelial NADPH oxidase [5]. However, we have recently shown that these oxidants produce relatively less damage than the oxidants of thalassemia major, as the lipid peroxidation marker malondialdehyde is elevated in the plasma of thalassemia more than in SCD, indicating that differences between SCD and thalassemia exist at the level of certain oxidant markers [6]. This may be due to the higher levels of non-transferrin-bound iron (NTBI) in thalassemia compared to SCD [6]. Sickle hemoglobin is also injurious to endothelial cells [7] and may contribute to the other makers characteristic to the pathophysiology of SCD that include leukocytosis, which results in increased production of damaging cytokines and altered blood flow, coagulation abnormalities, and abnormal vascular regulation. Previously, we also found differences between the inflammatory cytokine levels of SCD and thalassemia patients, with SCD patients having higher levels of IL-10 and IL-5 than thalassemia patients [6]. For SCD patients, the net result of these abnormalities is a shortened erythrocyte lifespan due to intravascular hemolysis, intermittent vascular occlusion, and chronic inflammation. Transfusion therapy is effective to treat the complications of the disease, with the vast majority of SCD patients having received transfusion therapy by adulthood. However, this results in damaging iron overload, which necessitates chelation therapy for control.

Basic Iron Metabolism in SCD

Iron Absorption

Iron entry and metabolism begins either at the gastrointestinal tract or by transfusion. With no known major physiologic pathway for iron excretion, absorption at the intestine has been found to be the primary site for regulating body iron stores [8]. The expression levels of genes that regulate iron absorption and metabolism differ depending on whether the iron burden is derived from increased iron absorption or through blood transfusion. In uncomplicated SCD and β-thalassemia intermedia, where regular transfusion therapy is unnecessary, there is evidence of iron overload caused by enhanced intestinal absorption, but more so in thalassemia intermedia than SCD [9]. The reasons for this have not been extensively studied, but it appears that SCD has less enhanced iron absorption than thalassemia [9] and SCD patients may also lose iron at a higher rate than in thalassemia. In thalassemia, iron absorption studies show that the rate of loading from the gastrointestinal tract is approximately three to four times greater than the normal rate [10], and higher than in SCD [9], although few studies have addressed this. Increased iron absorption also plays a role in the pathophysiology of β-thalassemia major, where it is inversely related to hemoglobin levels.

Non-heme iron (Fe^{3+} bound to bioorganic ligands in food) is the most abundant form of available dietary iron, but it is the least easily absorbed. Only 1–10% (depending on the type of dietary ligand) is taken up by the enterocytes in the duodenum and proximal jejunum. Heme iron is better absorbed, with 15–20% being absorbed through heme carrier protein 1 [11]. Recent work also implicates ferritin absorption in the gut [12]. For the absorption of non-heme iron, duodenal brush border cytochrome b reduces Fe^{3+} to Fe^{2+} for its transport into the enterocyte by divalent metal transporter 1 (DMT1) [13]. Molecular studies support ascorbate as the electron donor for duodenal ferri-reductase activity and provide role for ascorbate in intestinal iron absorption [14]. It has been suggested that patients with hemosiderosis should avoid excessive ascorbate intake to prevent further iron absorption [15] and possibly enhanced oxidant stress [16], although this has never been proven. However, a therapeutic use for ascorbate administration is called for when the ascorbate level is low, to increase urinary iron in combination with deferoxamine (DFO) chelation therapy [17]. DMT1 is a divalent metal transporter with broad substrate specificity, transporting Fe^{2+}, Zn^{2+}, Mn^{2+}, and other ions [18]. DMT1-mediated Fe^{2+} transport has been shown to be pH dependent and coupled to proton symport, which may explain why some patients treated with antacids have iron deficiency [19]. However, a few early studies indicated that SCD patients have no difference in their gastric acid secretions compared with normal controls [20]. Classical iron absorption studies in the 1960s and 1970s showed enhanced iron absorption in SCD [9, 21, 22]. Thus, DMT1 regulation may be modulated in SCD. For example, expression of DMT1 is dramatically induced in iron deficiency [23]. In support of the idea that

SCD may enhance DMT1 expression through iron deficiency, it has been shown that young SCD patients can be iron deficient [24] and may even require iron supplementation to initiate erythropoiesis [25]. Thus, it could be that in some young SCD patients with high erythropoietic drive DMT1 expression is enhanced.

Enhanced iron uptake in SCD could also be caused by iron loss through the urine as either heme or free iron [26]. SCD patients have intravascular hemolysis [27], while much of the hemolysis in thalassemia major is extravascular in the bone marrow. The contribution of this intravascular free hemoglobin to urinary iron is unclear. Examining 1 patient each with SCD, sickle thalassemia, and thalassemia major, Sears et al. [28] reported elevated urinary iron levels in all 3 patients with the greatest elevation in the SCD patient. The iron was characterized as predominantly 'insoluble iron' (hemosiderin) with negligible amounts in hemoglobin. This iron presumably arose from renal cells loaded with hemosiderin iron being sloughed into the urine. In addition, the same authors infused 19 g of hemoglobin in a normal individual as a control and demonstrated that most of the iron found in the urine was bound to hemoglobin, in contrast to the pattern seen in the patients with SCD or thalassemia. Based on this very limited report, it is difficult to suggest that elevated renal iron excretion in SCD is different from other hemoglobinopathies. In terms of renal deposition of iron, Schein et al. [29] have recently used MRI to demonstrate significantly enhanced renal iron deposits in SCD compared to thalassemia and control patients; these renal deposits were correlated with intravascular hemolysis. Washington and Boggs [26] provided a more extensive examination of urinary iron excretion in SCD showing elevation above normal in 27 of 31 patients, but did not compare SCD to other hemoglobinopathies. Also possible is that the kidney of SCD patients, which is prone to insufficiency, may be metabolizing more heme and/or iron in certain parts of the proximal and distal tubules as might also be inferred from recent animal studies [30–32]. Thus, part of the differences in iron trafficking between SCD and other hemoglobinopathies may take place in the kidney with more iron retention [29] or perhaps more release into the urine [26]. This may be due to renal insufficiency or a change in renal iron processing in SCD.

Iron absorption is completed by its release to transferrin through ferroportin (FPN) [33]. If FPN is the port or gate through which iron is released, the 'gatekeeper' is hepcidin. This 25-amino-acid hormone is synthesized in liver hepatocytes and has been found to control the release of iron at FPN by causing its internalization and degradation [34]. Extensive research on hepcidin has revealed that its expression is increased by hepatic iron [8] thereby reducing iron absorption. Hepcidin is also raised by the inflammatory cytokine IL-6 [35], controlling potential iron availability to pathogenic organisms, with chronic expression leading to the anemia of chronic disease [36]. Demand for iron in deficiency or in hypoxia-induced erythropoiesis decreases hepatic hepcidin production. Hypoxia may directly influence hepatocytes by increasing hypoxia-inducible factor 1 [37], or renal sensing of hypoxia, and the release of erythropoietin (EPO) may lower hepcidin [8]. Pediatric SCD patients have been found to have low levels of hepcidin [38, 39], perhaps induced by the hypoxia and/or anemia of SCD, which could then lead to the enhanced iron absorption found.

Many patients with SCD are cared for with transfusion (to prevent possible stroke and symptomatic anemia). This transfusional iron load increases hepatic hepcidin production [40], which reduces the enhanced intestinal iron uptake in SCD (and thalassemia), suppressing erythropoiesis [22]. Observations such as those discussed above have led to the conclusion that iron absorption is regulated by *hypoxia* (shared by both SCD and thalassemia) and *body iron level*. Erythropoiesis also regulates iron absorption and if it is ineffective, there will be enhanced iron absorption from the duodenum [8].

Erythropoietic Iron Metabolism

Erythropoietic activity is a tightly regulated process and is adjusted by the loss of red blood cells (RBCs) and renal vascular oxygen tension [41]. Normal bone marrow hematopoiesis produces approximately 10^{10} erythrocytes per hour to maintain hemoglobin levels within fairly narrow limits with production being rapidly increased with blood loss, RBC loss by hemolysis (or apoptosis of precursors), or hypoxia. Important factors leading to potential ineffective erythropoiesis (IE) in SCD (and thalassemia) are premature hemolysis of mature non-nucleated RBCs, apoptosis of erythroid precursors, and stalled erythroid differentiation [8].

The demand for erythropoiesis can control iron availability through four distinct cell types: (1) the iron-*absorbing* duodenal enterocytes, (2) the iron-*storing* hepatocytes, (3) the iron-*recycling* reticuloendothelial (RE) macrophages, and (4) the *oxygen-sensing* renal tubule epithelial cells. Two broad hormone systems control these four cell types to modulate iron levels in response to demand. First, as discussed above, hepcidin controls iron release through FPN at the basolateral membrane of duodenal cells, hepatocytes, and macrophages [42]. Thus hepcidin could be thought of as the 'gatekeeper' for iron in these cells. Furthermore, in spite of the high levels of IL-6 in non-transfused SCD patients, they still have low hepcidin levels, indicating that anemia or hypoxia has a strong influence on hepcidin expression.

Second, the erythroid drive that controls iron demand is most likely a combination of two cytokine-like hormones, growth differentiation factor 15 (GDF15) and EPO. GDF15 (also know as macrophage inhibitory cytokine-1) mRNA is most abundant in hepatocytes, with lower levels seen in some other tissues, especially the erythroid cells of the bone marrow. Expression of GDF15 in liver can be significantly up-regulated during injury to liver, kidney, heart, and lung, and this is mediated by IL-1β, TNFα, IL-2, M-CSF, TGFβ, and p53 [43–45]. However, the expanded erythroid compartment in hemoglobinopathies such as thalassemia secretes high levels of GDF15, which most likely leads to iron overload by its ability to *inhibit* hepcidin expression [46]. This recent work also found a non-significant elevation in the level of GDF15 in 13 SCD patients. Further research with more patients will reveal the role of GDF15 in SCD. Also, twisted gastrulation (TWSG1) may also be an erythroid regulator of hepcidin [47]. The levels of TWSG1 have not been investigated in SCD.

Lastly, concerning EPO metabolism, we would like to point out the possible importance of the kidney in the control of erythropoiesis and iron metabolism in SCD. The kidney is in a strategic position to sense both oxygen levels and iron load and could, in hemolytic anemias such as SCD, release iron and/or heme should the need arise. The relationship between EPO and hepcidin has recently been demonstrated, but the specific mechanisms that regulate prohepcidin renal expression in hemolytic anemia, a state with high EPO levels, are not known. It is possible that direct and/or indirect pathways are involved.

Bone Marrow Iron Metabolism

The bone marrow is a primary site of iron storage and RBC synthesis. In SCD and thalassemia, there is an expanded bone marrow and this also represents a site where iron storage problems associated with iron transport can exist. Usually, bone marrow RE macrophages are the primary site of iron storage in normal physiologic conditions. However, in the pathologic conditions experienced in transfused SCD or thalassemia patients, macrophage iron increases with recruitment of iron storage in endothelial cells of the sinusoids [48]. A dynamic relationship exists between erythroblasts and macrophage storage

iron. The transfer of storage iron to erythroblasts results in the normal maintenance of approximately 30–40% sideroblasts. Qualitative and quantitative examination of sideroblasts has been helpful in diagnosing pathologic conditions. While the normal marrow has approximately 30–50% sideroblasts, it is now known that inflammatory-induced IL-6 triggers macrophage hepcidin expression, which leads to an autocrine internalization of FPN resulting in blocked macrophage iron release [49] and decreased sideroblastic iron relative to RE iron. Classically, in hemoglobinopathies such as β-thalassemia, sideroblasts have increased iron in correlation with macrophage hemosiderin. While the amount and distribution of iron in the bone marrow of sickle cell patients have not been extensively studied, there are enough data to suggest a marked disturbance in iron transport and storage. In contrast to the expected increased bone marrow iron stores, Oluboyede et al. [50] reported that 68 of 85 bone marrow aspirates performed in SCD patients had absent marrow iron. In support of this, Rao et al. [51] found absent bone marrow iron or altered distribution in 25 children and young adults. This abnormality in bone marrow iron transport in SCD is supported by indirect laboratory tests for functional iron deficiencies. Vichinsky et al. [24] evaluated 70 sickle cell patients with laboratory tests including free erythrocyte protoporphyrin, serum ferritin, and serum transferrin saturation and found low levels of iron storage markers. An iron supplementation challenge was given to all patients regardless of the iron stores reflected in their laboratory tests. Surprisingly, in over 9% of all patients hemoglobin rose >2 g. This implies that iron stores in SCD are either quantitatively decreased or less mobilizable compared with oral iron. O'Brien [52] evaluated iron stores in SCD patients using DFO-induced excretion. His work found significantly less iron excretion in SCD relative to thalassemia, suggesting less stored iron in SCD, supporting the results of Vichinsky et al. [24].

Studies focusing on frequently transfused SCD patients further support evidence for a marked disturbance in iron deposition and transport in SCD. Normally, bone marrow iron studies from patients recurrently transfused demonstrate increased iron storage. While data are limited in chronically transfused SCD, these patients appear different from other transfused groups such as thalassemia patients. SCD patients with a history of recurrent transfusions do not show increased bone marrow iron [24] or large increases in NTBI [6]. Peterson et al. [25] performed bone marrow examinations in 39 SCD patients who had elevated serum ferritin levels with a history of transfusion. Surprisingly, one third of the patients had no stainable iron in the marrow despite elevated ferritin levels, supporting the hypothesis of a defect in iron transport. Autopsy studies, while limited, support these observations. In a study by Natta et al. [53], iron was totally absent in all organs in 1 adult SCD patient. In another study, marked iron overload was found in the liver, spleen, and kidney with complete absence of iron in the bone marrow despite elevated ferritin. Pippard et al. [54] have hypothesized that SCD patients have a significantly different clinical course compared with β-thalassemia patients because their iron stores remain locked in a nontoxic form in RE system macrophages longer than in β-thalassemia patients. In a 1994 review, the authors suggested that SCD patients may be at significantly less risk of iron overload because of the pathologic iron deposition induced by inflammation in SCD [55]. Unfortunately, definitive data for these suggestions have not yet been generated. It is also possible that the iron storage mechanism or trafficking in the bone marrow differs from that found in the liver or spleen or in response to the underlying disease.

Ferritin

The high levels of ferritin in transfused SCD and thalassemia patients is plausibly caused by iron that is preferentially distributed to the RE system and subsequent ferritin synthesis and release into the circulation. However, ferritin is an acute-phase protein and can be increased in inflammation, and SCD patients have high levels of circulating cytokines, IL-1, IL-6, and IL-10; indeed IL-1β elevates H- and L-ferritin subunit synthesis in both human hepatoma cells (HepG2) and primary human umbilical vein endothelial cells [56]; IL-6 also causes a moderate increase in L-subunit synthesis [56]. Furthermore, serum ferritin has been shown to be correlated with the inflammatory C-reactive protein in hemodialysis patients [57], and steady-state SCD patients have high levels of C-reactive protein [6] which increases further in crisis [58]. However, non-transfused SCD patients have only moderately elevated ferritin levels, thus the rise in ferritin in SCD could be due to a combination of factors including inflammation and iron retention in the RE system. Also, the disease or ethnic differences in the H-ferritin ferroxidase amount and activity may explain part of the specific iron metabolism in SCD [59].

Transferrin

In non-transfused SCD patients, the transferrin saturation is generally low, which is consistent with their ane-

mia; however, in transfused patients with SCD, transferrin saturations are similar to but not as high as those in transfused thalassemia major patients.

Transferrin is also modulated during inflammation by the immune system, with levels decreasing in inflammation [60] (which seems contradictory to its iron sequestration function). However, in line with the enhanced inflammatory levels in SCD, it has been found that transferrin levels are low in SCD [61].

Non-Transferrin-Bound Iron

The increase in NTBI most likely occurs when transferrin is saturated and possibly released from splenic macrophages recycling iron from senescent RBCs. Transfused SCD patients have increased NTBI [6] most likely from this recycling. NTBI is now recognized to consist of several components [62]: (a) directly chelatable iron, a fraction immediately accessible to chelators; (b) redox-active iron, and (c) redox-inactive iron. These species are likely to be interrelated and possibly interconvertible. There is evidence that some forms of NTBI are taken into cardiac myocytes and endocrine tissues through L-type calcium-dependent calcium channels [63]. These calcium channels are unevenly expressed on different tissues and may contribute to the differential tissue distribution of iron seen in chronic transfusional overload. However, little is known about how different components of NTBI are handled by these receptors. We have shown that total NTBI levels are lower in SCD patients than in thalassemia major [6]. We suggest that these differences are due to the inflammatory differences between the two groups.

Over time chronically transfused SCD patients may accumulate iron in the liver, and hepatocytes may be able to take up NTBI not described by the previously discussed mechanisms. However, the hepatocyte NTBI uptake mechanism has not been elucidated. Potential candidates are DMT1, ZIP14, and neutrophil gelatinase-associated lipocalin. Plasma levels of neutrophil gelatinase-associated lipocalin are enhanced in thalassemia [64], but have not been investigated in SCD.

RE System Macrophages and the Spleen

Splenic (and also liver) macrophages phagocytize senescent and damaged erythrocytes from the blood stream and then recycle the iron back to the bone marrow via transferrin. RBCs of SCD are fragile and have enhanced oxidants which cause them to age much faster; with normal erythrocytes circulating for 120 days, SCD erythrocytes circulate for a quarter of the time or less. Recent work shows that macrophage integrins can bind erythrocytes through ICAM-4 (CD242) and that phagocytosis of senescent erythrocytes is in part dependent on ICAM-4/β_2-integrin [65]. Also important is that macrophage recognition and phagocytosis is initiated by an abnormal translocation of phosphatidylserine in SCD erythrocytes [66]. Recent data have further shown that the increased phosphatidylserine exposure on these erythrocytes is induced by substances from activated neutrophils with which the less deformable sickle erythrocytes have close contact in narrow capillaries [67]. It is thus likely that removal of the senescent sickle erythrocytes is accelerated by exogenous factors, inducing phosphatidylserine exposure. Once the erythrocyte has been phagocytized it is catabolized in lysosomes and the heme is degraded by heme oxygenase-1 to yield ferrous iron. Heme oxygenase-1 is also an important anti-inflammatory enzyme that has been found to have enhanced expression in monocytes of sickle mice and in circulating endothelial cells of SCD patients, and has been found to play a role in the inhibition of vaso-occlusion [68]. Egress of iron from macrophages involves FPN [69]. Increased expression of DMT1 in inflammation occurs in macrophages and possibly in SCD [70].

Another protein that might be important in SCD and is capable of erythroid and macrophage heme export is feline leukemia virus, subgroup C receptor. This cell surface protein has been shown to export cytoplasmic heme, protect erythroid cells from heme toxicity, and be essential for erythropoiesis [71]. These results and recent findings suggest that erythroid precursors export excess toxic heme to ensure survival and that heme trafficking is a normal part of erythropoiesis and systemic iron balance [72].

However, in SCD inflammation may prevent iron release from storage sites, particularly macrophages, thereby decreasing transferrin saturation and iron transport to tissues with a high iron requirement such as the bone marrow. Only one study has examined RE system processing of transfused RBCs in humans [73]. Inflammation produced a blockade in the early phase of Fe release, possibly by inducing ferritin synthesis and cellular iron storage and increasing plasma hepcidin concentrations. Similarly, in vitro studies demonstrate that inflammation and cytokines stimulate the uptake and retention of iron in monocytes and RE cells [74]. As described above, hepcidin has been shown to prevent iron egress from cells in culture by complexing with FPN and inducing its internalization [34]. This multifunctional iron regulator is induced by IL-1 and IL-6 [75], further linking inflammation to iron stores and regulation. In a recent publication, hepcidin was identified as being synthesized in circulating monocyte cells, suggesting an autocrine function of this important regulatory molecule [76].

Hepatocyte Iron Regulation

Hepatic hepcidin expression is generally decreased in iron deficiency anemia, hypoxia, and IE and increased in inflammatory states [8]. The relationship of hepcidin synthesis to iron metabolism and iron overload is less clear. In tissue culture, transferrin saturation appears to positively regulate hepcidin synthesis [77] whereas NTBI may have opposite effects both in vitro [78] and in thalassemia major patients [79]. In patients with hemoglobinopathies, urinary hepcidin was increased in 3 patients with transfusional iron overload (2 patients with SCD and 1 with myelodysplastic syndrome) [78]. In contrast, no correlation was found between hepcidin and liver iron in thalassemia major patients, and an inverse correlation was noted with NTBI [79]. In congenital chronic anemia, urinary hepcidin was decreased and inversely correlated with erythropoietic drive. Although anemic patients with SCD without iron overload had low levels of urinary hepcidin [38], the effect of transfusion has not been studied in SCD patients. IE in thalassemia intermedia appears to be associated with decreased hepcidin synthesis in the liver compared with thalassemia major patients at matched levels of body iron loading [40]. A possible mechanism for inhibition of hepcidin synthesis in IE is GDF15 [46]. GDF15 is a hypoxia-driven factor which is markedly increased in the plasma of patients with β-thalassemia syndromes and appears to down-regulate hepcidin expression in hepatocytes. Down-regulation of hepcidin synthesis by IE, mediated through GDF15, may be the mechanism for increased iron absorption seen in syndromes associated with IE.

Role of Blood Transfusions in SCD

In 1998, the stroke prevention trial (STOP1) showed that the frequency of first stroke in children with SCD could be dramatically decreased with transfusion therapy [87]. Since that time, transfusions have been shown to also reduce the likelihood of acute chest syndrome, painful events, and growth failure [80]. Thus the use of transfusion therapy in SCD contrasts its use in thalassemia major, where transfusions are life sustaining [17]. Prevention of complications from stroke is the most common reason for starting transfusion in SCD and can reduce the risk of repeated stroke from approximately 70 to 10–20% [81].

Iron Overload and Chelation in SCD

Iron overload secondary to transfusion therapy is a common problem in SCD; 90% of patients have received transfusion therapy by adulthood. Many SCD patients are inadequately screened and treated for hemosiderosis. In contrast to thalassemia patients, they receive intermittent transfusions. These patients often do not receive comprehensive hemosiderosis screening and treatment.

Iron overload requires treatment in SCD. There are two methods to decrease iron overload in transfused patients. Red cell pheresis instead of simple transfusion dramatically decreases the iron burden and delays or prevents the need for chelation therapy. However, this technique is expensive, invasive, and not readily available. Most patients, therefore, require the use of chelation to control iron overload. There are three methods to determine when chelation therapy should be initiated and modified. Optimally, all three methods should be utilized in the monitoring of iron overload in SCD. Quantitative assessment of liver iron is a reliable indicator of body iron stores; it can be determined by liver biopsy, magnetic resonance, or ferritometer. Chelation therapy should be initiated when the liver iron reaches 3,000 μg/g dry weight. Serum ferritin is affected by inflammation and is less reliable in SCD. In the steady state, a serum ferritin >1,000 ng/ml suggests chelation therapy is indicated. It should be paired with another indicator. The transfusion burden is a useful and reliable indicator of iron overload. Patients receiving >120 ml packed RBCs/kg body weight or >1 year of monthly transfusions are likely to require chelation therapy.

There are three clinically available iron chelators: DFO, deferiprone (L1), and deferasirox (Exjade). DFO is the most studied iron chelator and has an excellent safety and efficacy profile. Its poor oral bioavailability and short half-life requires subcutaneous or intravenous administration 8–12 h daily, 5–7 days per week. While efficacious, DFO use is limited by poor compliance and local reactions [17].

Exjade (ICL670, deferasirox) is a once-daily, orally absorbed tridentate iron chelator that binds iron in a 2:1 ratio. It is absorbed rapidly and reaches a peak plasma level within 1–3 h. Iron excretion occurs almost exclusively through the fecal route. Also, in studies examining plasma NTBI and its toxic counterpart, labile plasma iron, Exjade has been shown to decrease NTBI and labile plasma iron in patients with transfusional iron overload [82]. This may be due to the enhanced plasma half-life of Exjade compared to DFO. It has been found to be efficacious in the treatment of iron overload in SCD trials [83].

In general, deferasirox appears similar to DFO in lowering iron and serum ferritin in a dose-dependent manner. The starting dose of Exjade is at least 20 mg/kg/day. Higher doses of 30 mg/kg/day may be required to establish a negative iron balance. Patients with SCD have been reported to be more satisfied with the use of Exjade and to have an improved quality of life compared to DFO [84]. Deferasirox toxicities include skin rash, nausea, and diarrhea; these are often transient. In SCD, potential renal complications from deferasirox require close monitoring of creatinine. There is no evidence that sickle cell patients have increased renal dysfunction from deferasirox. However, since sickle cell patients have a high risk of renal failure, long-term studies with deferasirox are indicated.

Deferiprone (L1/Ferriprox) is approved for use in several countries, but not the United States. Deferiprone reduces or maintains total body iron stores in the majority of patients, and appears to be superior to DFO in removing cardiac iron. Studies in SCD are very limited. The standard therapeutic daily dose is 75 mg/kg three times daily. The major side effects of deferiprone include gastrointestinal symptoms, joint pain, and neutropenia. While uncommon, agranulocytosis has resulted in rare deaths. Therefore, weekly white blood cell counts are required for all patients receiving deferiprone. Similar to Exjade, zinc deficiency may be increased in SCD.

Conclusions and Summary

Recent data showing that hepcidin is low in non-transfused pediatric SCD patients are consistent with classic iron absorption studies that demonstrated increased iron absorption in SCD. In contrast, transfused SCD adults have been found to have increased hepcidin levels suggesting that iron burden and inflammation in combination with reduced anemia/hypoxia leads to the increased hepcidin. Interestingly, SCD patients lose iron faster than other hemoglobinopathy patients and this may be related to iron deposition in the kidney or urine. SCD patients also have lower NTBI levels compared with other hemoglobinopathies such as thalassemia, which may be linked to the decreased frequency of iron deposition in the heart found in thalassemia. Care for SCD now commonly uses regular RBC transfusions that result in heavy iron overload and necessitate the need for chelation therapy. New oral chelation using deferasirox appears to be safe and may even lower the amount of toxic free NTBI and increase patient compliance. Finally, we suggest that iron metabolism and trafficking is different in SCD compared to other hemoglobinopathies and that the high levels of inflammatory cytokines enhance either macrophage RE cell iron retention or renal iron retention, which may protect these patients from organ failure seen in other hemoglobinopathies such as the cardiomyopathy and endocrine failure seen in thalassemia.

Acknowledgments

The authors would like to thank Ward Hagar, David Killilea, Fernando Viteri, and Claudia Morris for reviewing their areas of expertise and making valuable corrections and suggestions.

References

1 Konotey-Ahulu FID: Effect of environment on sickle cell disease in West Africa: Epidemiologic and clinical considerations; in Abramson H, Bertles JF, Wethers DL (eds): Sickle Cell Disease, Diagnosis, Management, Education and Research. St. Louis, Mosby, 1973, p 20.

2 Modell B, Darlison M: Global epidemiology of haemoglobin disorders and derived service indicators. Bull World Health Organ 2008;86:480–487.

3 Repka T, Hebbel RP: Hydroxyl radical formation by sickle erythrocyte membranes: role of pathologic iron deposits and cytoplasmic reducing agents. Blood 1991;78:2753–2758.

4 Aslan M, Freeman BA: Oxidant-mediated impairment of nitric oxide signaling in sickle cell disease – mechanisms and consequences. Cell Mol Biol (Noisy-le-grand) 2004;50:95–105.

5 Wood KC, Hebbel RP, Granger DN: Endothelial cell NADPH oxidase mediates the cerebral microvascular dysfunction in sickle cell transgenic mice. FASEB J 2005;19:989–991.

6 Walter PB, Fung EB, Killilea DW, Jiang Q, Hudes M, Madden J, Porter J, Evans P, Vichinsky E, Harmatz P: Oxidative stress and inflammation in iron-overloaded patients with beta-thalassaemia or sickle cell disease. Br J Haematol 2006;135:254–263.

7 Hebbel RP: Blockade of adhesion of sickle cells to endothelium by monoclonal antibodies. N Engl J Med 2000;342:1910–1912.

8 Rechavi G, Rivella S: Regulation of iron absorption in hemoglobinopathies. Curr Mol Med 2008;8:646–662.

9 Erlandson ME, Walden B, Stern G, Hilgartner MW, Wehman J, Smith CH: Studies on congenital hemolytic syndromes, IV. Gastrointestinal absorption of iron. Blood 1962; 19:359–378.

10 Olivieri NF: Progression of iron overload in sickle cell disease. Semin Hematol 2001;38: 57–62.

11 Shayeghi M, Latunde-Dada GO, Oakhill JS, Laftah AH, Takeuchi K, Halliday N, Khan Y, Warley A, McCann FE, Hider RC, Frazer DM, Anderson GJ, Vulpe CD, Simpson RJ, McKie AT: Identification of an intestinal heme transporter. Cell 2005;122:789–801.

12 Lonnerdal B, Bryant A, Liu X, Theil EC: Iron absorption from soybean ferritin in nonanemic women. Am J Clin Nutr 2006;83:103–107.

13 Latunde-Dada GO, Van der Westhuizen J, Vulpe CD, Anderson GJ, Simpson RJ, McKie AT: Molecular and functional roles of duodenal cytochrome b (Dcytb) in iron metabolism. Blood Cells Mol Dis 2002;29:356–360.

14 Atanassova BD, Tzatchev KN: Ascorbic acid – important for iron metabolism. Folia Med (Plovdiv) 2008;50:11–16.

15 Mallory MA, Sthapanachai C, Kowdley KV: Iron overload related to excessive vitamin C intake. Ann Intern Med 2003;139:532–533.

16 Nienhuis AW: Vitamin C and iron. N Engl J Med 1981;304:170–171.

17 Kwiatkowski JL, Cohen AR: Iron chelation therapy in sickle-cell disease and other transfusion-dependent anemias. Hematol Oncol Clin North Am 2004;18:1355–1377, ix.

18 Picard V, Govoni G, Jabado N, Gros P: Nramp 2 (DCT1/DMT1) expressed at the plasma membrane transports iron and other divalent cations into a calcein-accessible cytoplasmic pool. J Biol Chem 2000;275:35738–35745.

19 Andrews NC: Forging a field: the golden age of iron biology. Blood 2008;112:219–230.

20 Lee MG, Thirumalai CH, Terry SI, Serjeant GR: Endoscopic and gastric acid studies in homozygous sickle cell disease and upper abdominal pain. Gut 1989;30:569–572.

21 Ringelhann B, Konotey-Ahulu F, Dodu SR: Studies on iron metabolism in sickle cell anaemia, sickle cell haemoglobin C disease, and haemoglobin C disease using a large volume liquid scintillation counter. J Clin Pathol 1970;23:127–134.

22 Erlandson ME, Schulman I, Smith CH: Studies on congenital hemolytic syndromes. III. Rates of destruction and production of erythrocytes in sickle cell anemia. Pediatrics 1960;25:629–644.

23 Gunshin H, Mackenzie B, Berger UV, Gunshin Y, Romero MF, Boron WF, Nussberger S, Gollan JL, Hediger MA: Cloning and characterization of a mammalian proton-coupled metal-ion transporter. Nature 1997;388: 482–488.

24 Vichinsky E, Kleman K, Embury S, Lubin B: The diagnosis of iron deficiency anemia in sickle cell disease. Blood 1981;58:963–968.

25 Peterson CM, Graziano JH, de Ciutiis A, Grady RW, Cerami A, Worwood M, Jacobs A: Iron metabolism, sickle cell disease, and response to cyanate. Blood 1975;46:583–590.

26 Washington R, Boggs DR: Urinary iron in patients with sickle cell anemia. J Lab Clin Med 1975;86:17–23.

27 Kato GJ, McGowan V, Machado RF, Little JA, Taylor JT, Morris CR, Nichols JS, Wang X, Poljakovic M, Morris SM Jr, Gladwin MT: Lactate dehydrogenase as a biomarker of hemolysis-associated nitric oxide resistance, priapism, leg ulceration, pulmonary hypertension, and death in patients with sickle cell disease. Blood 2006;107:2279–2285.

28 Sears DA, Anderson PR, Foy AL, Williams HL, Crosby WH: Urinary iron excretion and renal metabolism of hemoglobin in hemolytic diseases. Blood 1966;28:708–725.

29 Schein A, Enriquez C, Coates TD, Wood JC: Magnetic resonance detection of kidney iron deposition in sickle cell disease: a marker of chronic hemolysis. J Magn Reson Imaging 2008;28:698–704.

30 Kulaksiz H, Theilig F, Bachmann S, Gehrke SG, Rost D, Janetzko A, Cetin Y, Stremmel W: The iron-regulatory peptide hormone hepcidin: expression and cellular localization in the mammalian kidney. J Endocrinol 2005;184:361–370.

31 Veuthey T, D'Anna MC, Roque ME: Role of the kidney in iron homeostasis: renal expression of prohepcidin, ferroportin, and DMT1 in anemic mice. Am J Physiol Renal Physiol 2008;295:F1213–F1221.

32 Wareing M, Ferguson CJ, Delannoy M, Cox AG, McMahon RF, Green R, Riccardi D, Smith CP: Altered dietary iron intake is a strong modulator of renal DMT1 expression. Am J Physiol Renal Physiol 2003;285:F1050–F1059.

33 Donovan A, Brownlie A, Zhou Y, Shepard J, Pratt SJ, Moynihan J, Paw BH, Drejer A, Barut B, Zapata A, Law TC, Brugnara C, Lux SE, Pinkus GS, Pinkus JL, Kingsley PD, Palis J, Fleming MD, Andrews NC, Zon LI: Positional cloning of zebrafish ferroportin1 identifies a conserved vertebrate iron exporter. Nature 2000;403:776–781.

34 Nemeth E, Tuttle MS, Powelson J, Vaughn MB, Donovan A, Ward DM, Ganz T, Kaplan J: Hepcidin regulates cellular iron efflux by binding to ferroportin and inducing its internalization. Science 2004;306:2090–2093.

35 Nemeth E, Rivera S, Gabayan V, Keller C, Taudorf S, Pedersen BK, Ganz T: IL-6 mediates hypoferremia of inflammation by inducing the synthesis of the iron regulatory hormone hepcidin. J Clin Invest 2004;113:1271–1276.

36 Weiss G: Iron metabolism in the anemia of chronic disease. Biochim Biophys Acta 2009;1790:682–693.

37 Peyssonnaux C, Zinkernagel AS, Schuepbach RA, Rankin E, Vaulont S, Haase VH, Nizet V, Johnson RS: Regulation of iron homeostasis by the hypoxia-inducible transcription factors (HIFs). J Clin Invest 2007;117:1926–1932.

38 Kearney SL, Nemeth E, Neufeld EJ, Thapa D, Ganz T, Weinstein DA, Cunningham MJ: Urinary hepcidin in congenital chronic anemias. Pediatr Blood Cancer 2007;48:57–63.

39 Kroot JJ, Laarakkers CM, Kemna EH, Biemond BJ, Swinkels DW: Regulation of serum hepcidin levels in sickle cell disease. Haematologica 2009;94:885–887.

40 Origa R, Galanello R, Ganz T, Giagu N, Maccioni L, Faa G, Nemeth E: Liver iron concentrations and urinary hepcidin in beta-thalassemia. Haematologica 2007;92:583–588.

41 Eckardt KU: Erythropoietin: oxygen-dependent control of erythropoiesis and its failure in renal disease. Nephron 1994;67:7–23.

42 Nemeth E: Iron regulation and erythropoiesis. Curr Opin Hematol 2008;15:169–175.

43 Ago T, Sadoshima J: GDF15, a cardioprotective TGF-beta superfamily protein. Circ Res 2006;98:294–297.

44 Hsiao EC, Koniaris LG, Zimmers-Koniaris T, Sebald SM, Huynh TV, Lee SJ: Characterization of growth-differentiation factor 15, a transforming growth factor beta superfamily member induced following liver injury. Mol Cell Biol 2000;20:3742–3751.

45 Zimmers TA, Jin X, Hsiao EC, McGrath SA, Esquela AF, Koniaris LG: Growth differentiation factor-15/macrophage inhibitory cytokine-1 induction after kidney and lung injury. Shock 2005;23:543–548.

46 Tanno T, Bhanu NV, Oneal PA, Goh SH, Staker P, Lee YT, Moroney JW, Reed CH, Luban NL, Wang RH, Eling TE, Childs R, Ganz T, Leitman SF, Fucharoen S, Miller JL: High levels of GDF15 in thalassemia suppress expression of the iron regulatory protein hepcidin. Nat Med 2007;13:1096–1101.

47 Tanno T, Porayette P, Sripichai O, Noh SJ, Byrnes C, Bhupatiraju A, Lee YT, Goodnough JB, Harandi O, Ganz T, Paulson RF, Miller JL: Identification of TWSG1 as a second novel erythroid regulator of hepcidin expression in murine and human cells. Blood 2009;114:181–186.

48 Dullmann J, Wulfhekel U: Differences in the pattern of iron accumulation in primary and secondary hemochromatosis. Diagnostic importance and clinical consequences (in German). Folia Haematol Int Mag Klin Morphol Blutforsch 1990;117:413–417.

49 Theurl I, Aigner E, Theurl M, Nairz M, Seifert M, Schroll A, Sonnweber T, Eberwein L, Witcher DR, Murphy AT, Wroblewski VJ, Wurz E, Datz C, Weiss G: Regulation of iron homeostasis in anemia of chronic disease and iron deficiency anemia: diagnostic and therapeutic implications. Blood 2009;113:5277–5286.

50 Oluboyede OA, Ajayi OA, Adeyokunnu AA: Iron studies in patients with sickle cell disease. Afr J Med Med Sci 1981;10:1–7.

51 Rao KR, Patel AR, Honig GR, Vida LN, McGinnis PR: Iron deficiency and sickle cell anemia. Arch Intern Med 1983;143:1030–1032.

52 O'Brien RT: Iron burden in sickle cell anemia. J Pediatr 1978;92:579–582.

53 Natta C, Creque L, Navarro C: Compartmentalization of iron in sickle cell anemia – an autopsy study. Am J Clin Pathol 1985;83:76–78.

54 Pippard MJ: Iron overload and iron chelation therapy in thalassaemia and sickle cell haemoglobinopathies. Acta Haematol 1987;78:206–211.

55 Pippard MJ: Secondary iron overload; in Brock JH, Halliday JW, Pippard MJ (eds): Iron Metabolism in Health and Disease. London, Saunders, 1994, pp 272–300.

56 Rogers JT: Ferritin translation by interleukin-1 and interleukin-6: the role of sequences upstream of the start codons of the heavy and light subunit genes. Blood 1996;87:2525–2537.

57 Kalantar-Zadeh K, Rodriguez RA, Humphreys MH: Association between serum ferritin and measures of inflammation, nutrition and iron in haemodialysis patients. Nephrol Dial Transplant 2004;19:141–149.

58 Bargoma EM, Mitsuyoshi JK, Larkin SK, Styles LA, Kuypers FA, Test ST: Serum C-reactive protein parallels secretory phospholipase A2 in sickle cell disease patients with vasoocclusive crisis or acute chest syndrome. Blood 2005;105:3384–3385.

59 Hagar W, Vichinsky EP, Theil EC: Liver ferritin subunit ratios in neonatal hemochromatosis. Pediatr Hematol Oncol 2003;20:229–235.

60 Ritchie RF, Palomaki GE, Neveux LM, Navolotskaia O, Ledue TB, Craig WY: Reference distributions for the negative acute-phase serum proteins, albumin, transferrin and transthyretin: a practical, simple and clinically relevant approach in a large cohort. J Clin Lab Anal 1999;13:273–279.

61 Hedo CC, Aken'ova YA, Okpala IE, Durojaiye AO, Salimonu LS: Acute phase reactants and severity of homozygous sickle cell disease. J Intern Med 1993;233:467–470.

62 Evans RW, Rafique R, Zarea A, Rapisarda C, Cammack R, Evans PJ, Porter JB, Hider RC: Nature of non-transferrin-bound iron: studies on iron citrate complexes and thalassemic sera. J Biol Inorg Chem 2008;13:57–74.

63 Oudit GY, Trivieri MG, Khaper N, Liu PP, Backx PH: Role of l-type Ca^{2+} channels in iron transport and iron-overload cardiomyopathy. J Mol Med 2006;84:349–364.

64 Roudkenar MH, Halabian R, Oodi A, Roushandeh AM, Yaghmai P, Najar MR, Amirizadeh N, Shokrgozar MA: Upregulation of neutrophil gelatinase-associated lipocalin, NGAL/Lcn2, in beta-thalassemia patients. Arch Med Res 2008;39:402–407.

65 Toivanen A, Ihanus E, Mattila M, Lutz HU, Gahmberg CG: Importance of molecular studies on major blood groups – intercellular adhesion molecule-4, a blood group antigen involved in multiple cellular interactions. Biochim Biophys Acta 2008;1780:456–466.

66 Kuypers FA, Yuan J, Lewis RA, Snyder LM, Kiefer CR, Bunyaratvej A, Fucharoen S, Ma L, Styles L, de Jong K, Schrier SL: Membrane phospholipid asymmetry in human thalassemia. Blood 1998;91:3044–3051.

67 Haynes J Jr, Obiako B, King JA, Hester RB, Ofori-Acquah S: Activated neutrophil-mediated sickle red blood cell adhesion to lung vascular endothelium: role of phosphatidylserine-exposed sickle red blood cells. Am J Physiol Heart Circ Physiol 2006;291:H1679–H1685.

68 Belcher JD, Mahaseth H, Welch TE, Otterbein LE, Hebbel RP, Vercellotti GM: Heme oxygenase-1 is a modulator of inflammation and vaso-occlusion in transgenic sickle mice. J Clin Invest 2006;116:808–816.

69 Knutson MD, Oukka M, Koss LM, Aydemir F, Wessling-Resnick M: Iron release from macrophages after erythrophagocytosis is up-regulated by ferroportin 1 overexpression and down-regulated by hepcidin. Proc Natl Acad Sci USA 2005;102:1324–1328.

70 Wang X, Garrick MD, Yang F, Dailey LA, Piantadosi CA, Ghio AJ: TNF, IFN-gamma, and endotoxin increase expression of DMT1 in bronchial epithelial cells. Am J Physiol Lung Cell Mol Physiol 2005;289:L24–L33.

71 Quigley JG, Yang Z, Worthington MT, Phillips JD, Sabo KM, Sabath DE, Berg CL, Sassa S, Wood BL, Abkowitz JL: Identification of a human heme exporter that is essential for erythropoiesis. Cell 2004;118:757–766.

72 Keel SB, Doty RT, Yang Z, Quigley JG, Chen J, Knoblaugh S, Kingsley PD, De Domenico I, Vaughn MB, Kaplan J, Palis J, Abkowitz JL: A heme export protein is required for red blood cell differentiation and iron homeostasis. Science 2008;319:825–828.

73 Fillet G, Beguin Y, Baldelli L: Model of reticuloendothelial iron metabolism in humans: abnormal behavior in idiopathic hemochromatosis and in inflammation. Blood 1989;74:844–851.

74 Ludwiczek S, Aigner E, Theurl I, Weiss G: Cytokine-mediated regulation of iron transport in human monocytic cells. Blood 2003; 101:4148–4154.

75 Lee P, Peng H, Gelbart T, Wang L, Beutler E: Regulation of hepcidin transcription by interleukin-1 and interleukin-6. Proc Natl Acad Sci USA 2005;102:1906–1910.

76 Theurl I, Theurl M, Seifert M, Mair S, Nairz M, Rumpold H, Zoller H, Bellmann-Weiler R, Niederegger H, Talasz H, Weiss G: Autocrine formation of hepcidin induces iron retention in human monocytes. Blood 2008; 111:2392–2399.

77 Lin L, Valore EV, Nemeth E, Goodnough JB, Gabayan V, Ganz T: Iron transferrin regulates hepcidin synthesis in primary hepatocyte culture through hemojuvelin and BMP2/4. Blood 2007;110:2182–2189.

78 Nemeth E, Valore EV, Territo M, Schiller G, Lichtenstein A, Ganz T: Hepcidin, a putative mediator of anemia of inflammation, is a type II acute-phase protein. Blood 2003;101: 2461–2463.

79 Kattamis A, Papassotiriou I, Palaiologou D, Apostolakou F, Galani A, Ladis V, Sakellaropoulos N, Papanikolaou G: The effects of erythropoetic activity and iron burden on hepcidin expression in patients with thalassemia major. Haematologica 2006;91:809–812.

80 Wang WC, Morales KH, Scher CD, Styles L, Olivieri N, Adams R, Brambilla D: Effect of long-term transfusion on growth in children with sickle cell anemia: results of the STOP trial. J Pediatr 2005;147:244–247.

81 Pegelow CH, Adams RJ, McKie V, Abboud M, Berman B, Miller ST, Olivieri N, Vichinsky E, Wang W, Brambilla D: Risk of recurrent stroke in patients with sickle cell disease treated with erythrocyte transfusions. J Pediatr 1995;126:896–899.

82 Daar S, Pathare A, Nick H, Kriemler-Krahn U, Hmissi A, Habr D, Taher A: Reduction in labile plasma iron during treatment with deferasirox, a once-daily oral iron chelator, in heavily iron-overloaded patients with beta-thalassaemia. Eur J Haematol 2009;82:454–457.

83 Vichinsky E, Onyekwere O, Porter J, Swerdlow P, Eckman J, Lane P, Files B, Hassell K, Kelly P, Wilson F, Bernaudin F, Forni GL, Okpala I, Ressayre-Djaffer C, Alberti D, Holland J, Marks P, Fung E, Fischer R, Mueller BU, Coates T: A randomised comparison of deferasirox versus deferoxamine for the treatment of transfusional iron overload in sickle cell disease. Br J Haematol 2007;136: 501–508.

84 Vichinsky E, Pakbaz Z, Onyekwere O, Porter J, Swerdlow P, Coates T, Lane P, Files B, Mueller BU, Coic L, Forni GL, Fischer R, Marks P, Rofail D, Abetz L, Baladi JF: Patient-reported outcomes of deferasirox (Exjade, ICL670) versus deferoxamine in sickle cell disease patients with transfusional hemosiderosis. Substudy of a randomized open-label phase II trial. Acta Haematol 2008;119:133–141.

85 Herrick JB: Peculiar elongated and sickle-shaped red blood corpuscle in a case of severe anemia. Arch Intern Med 1910;5:517–521.

86 Pauling L, Itano HA, Singer SJ, Wells IC: Sickle cell anemia, a molecular disease. Science 1949;110:543–548.

87 Adams RJ, McKie VC, Hsu L, Files B, Vichinsky E, Pegelow C, Abboud M, Gallagher D, Kutlar A, Nichols FT, Bonds DR, Brambilla D: Prevention of a first stroke by transfusions in children with sickle cell anemia and abnormal results on transcranial Doppler ultrasonography. N Engl J Med 1998;339:5–11.

Author Index Vol. 122, No. 2–3, 2009

Acta Haematologica

Subject Index Vol. 122, No. 2–3, 2009

KARGER

© 2009 S. Karger AG, Basel

Fax +41 61 306 12 34
E-Mail karger@karger.ch
www.karger.com

Accessible online at:
www.karger.com/aha

American Association of Blood Banks

Code of Federal Regulations, Title 21, Parts 800 to 1299

Food and Drugs, Revised as of April 1, 2008

Hematology, Transfusion Medicine

Contents

Explanation

Title 21:
- Chapter I – Food and Drug Administration, Department of Health and Human Services (Continued)

Subchapter H – Medical Devices
- General
- Labeling
- Medical device reporting
- Medical devices; reports of corrections and removals
- Establishment registration and device listing for manufacturers and initial importers of devices
- Exemptions from Federal pre-emption of State and local medical device requirements
- In vitro diagnostic products for human use
- Medical device recall authority
- Investigational device exemptions
- Premarket approval of medical devices
- Quality system regulation
- Medical device tracking requirements
- Postmarket surveillance
- Medical device classification procedures
- Procedures for performance standards development
- Clinical chemistry and clinical toxicology devices
- Hematology and pathology devices

- Immunology and microbiology devices
- Anesthesiology devices
- Cardiovascular devices
- Dental devices
- Ear, nose, and throat devices
- Gastroenterology-urology devices
- General and plastic surgery devices
- General hospital and personal use devices
- Neurological devices
- Obstetrical and gynaecological devices
- Ophthalmic devices
- Orthopedic devices
- Physical medicine devices
- Radiology devices
- Banned devices
- Performance standard for electrode lead wires and patient cables

Subchapter I – Mammography Quality Standards Act
- Mammography

Subchapter J – Radiological Health
- General
- Records and reports
- Notification of defects or failure to comply
- Repurchase, repairs, or replacement of electronic products
- Importation of electronic products

- Performance standards for electronic products; General
- Performance standards for ionizing radiation emitting products
- Performance standards for microwave and radio frequency emitting products
- Performance standards for light-emitting products
- Performance standards for sonic, infrasonic, and ultrasonic radiation-emitting products

Subchapter L – Regulations under certain other Acts administered by the Food and Drug Administration
- Regulations under the Federal Import Milk Act
- Regulations under the Federal Caustic Poison Act
- Control of communicable diseases
- Interstate conveyance sanitation
- Human tissue intended for transplantation
- Human cells, tissues, and cellular and tissue-based products

www.karger.com

KI 09241

Code of Federal Regulations, Title 21, Parts 800 to 1299
X + 786 p., 2 fig., 9 tab., soft cover, 2009
CHF 277.– / EUR 198.–
Prices subject to change
EUR price for Germany only
ISBN 978–3–8055–9279–6
Distributed in USA/Canada exclusively by the AABB, Bethesda, Md.

Basic selling price determined by the AABB

Order Form

Please send: _____ copy/ies

Postage and handling free with prepayment

Payment:
Please charge to my credit card
- ☐ American Express ☐ Diners ☐ Eurocard
- ☐ MasterCard ☐ Visa

Card No.: _____

Exp. date: _____

CVV/CVC _____
(3 digits in the signature field on the back of Visa and MasterCard)

☐ Check enclosed ☐ Please bill me

Orders may be placed with any bookshop, subscription agency, directly with the publisher or through a Karger distributor.

Fax: +41 61 306 12 34

S. Karger AG, P.O. Box, CH–4009 Basel (Switzerland)
E-Mail orders@karger.ch, **www.karger.com**

Name/Address:
_____
_____
_____
_____

Date: _____

Signature: _____

KARGER

A comprehensive color manual

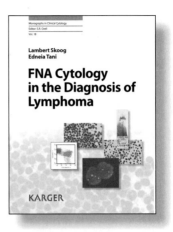

Lambert Skoog
Edneia Tani

FNA Cytology in the Diagnosis of Lymphoma

Cytology, Oncology, Pathology, Hematology

Main Headings

Fine-needle aspiration (FNA) became important for the cytology of the enlarged lymph node in the 1950s and 1960s and was accepted in the diagnosis of various types of lymphadenitis and metastatic disease. The diagnosis of lymphoma by FNA cytology, however, remained controversial for many years, as FNA smears did not allow the evaluation of growth pattern. Only later with the introduction of immunocytochemistry on FNA material it became possible to conclusively diagnose the majority of lymphomas with an accuracy comparable to that of histopathology. Other ancillary techniques such as FISH and PCR can now also be applied successfully to FNA material. These facts together with the excellent clinical performance of FNA sampling should increase the spread of the technique.

This comprehensive manual presents the cytomorphologic and immunocytochemical characteristics of both non-Hodgkin and Hodgkin lymphomas. It discusses the technical, methodological aspects of lymphoma diagnosis and describes the cytologic features of reactive lymphoid lesions and the major types of neoplastic lymphoid lesions, based on the most recent (2001) WHO lymphoma classification. Key cytologic and immunologic features are listed to facilitate a conclusive diagnosis of the different lesions.

This publication will be of immense value to clinicians such as cytopathologists, pathologists, oncologists, and hematologists involved in the clinical work-up and management of patients with lymph node lesions.

www.karger.com

KI 08228

Monographs in Clinical Cytology, Vol. 18
Series Editor: Orell, S.R. (Kent Town)
ISSN 0077–0809 / e-ISSN 1662–3827

Skoog, L.; Tani, E. (Stockholm)
FNA Cytology in the Diagnosis of Lymphoma
In collaboration with A. Porwit (Stockholm)
X + 78 p., 66 fig., 65 in color, 8 tab., hard cover, 2009
CHF 132.– / EUR 94.50 / USD 132.00
Prices subject to change
EUR price for Germany, USD price for USA only
ISBN 978–3–8055–8626–9
e-ISBN 978–3–8055–8627–6

Order Form

Please send: _____ copy/ies

Postage and handling free with prepayment

Payment:
Please charge to my credit card
☐ American Express   ☐ Diners   ☐ Eurocard
☐ MasterCard   ☐ Visa

Card No.: _____

Exp. date: _____

CVV/CVC _____
(3 digits in the signature field on the back of VISA and MasterCard)

☐ Check enclosed   ☐ Please bill me

Orders may be placed with any bookshop, subscription agency, directly with the publisher or through a Karger distributor.

Fax: +41 61 306 12 34

S. Karger AG, P.O. Box, CH–4009 Basel (Switzerland)
E-Mail orders@karger.ch, **www.karger.com**

Name/Address:

_____

_____

_____

_____

Date: _____

Signature: _____

KARGER